Instructor's Manual And Test Bank

for

Plowman • Smith

EXERCISE PHYSIOLOGY
for Health, Fitness, and Performance

prepared by

Sharon A. Plowman
Northern Illinois University

Denise L. Smith
Skidmore College

Patricia C. Fehling
Skidmore College

Allyn and Bacon
Boston · London · Toronto · Sydney · Tokyo · Singapore

Copyright © 1997 by Allyn & Bacon
A Viacom Company
160 Gould Street
Needham Heights, Massachusetts 02194

Internet: www.abacon.com
America Online: keyword: College Online

All rights reserved. The contents, or parts thereof, may be reproduced for use with *Exercise Physiology for Health, Fitness, and Performance,* by Sharon A. Plowman and Denise L. Smith, provided such reproductions bear copyright notice, but may not be reproduced in any form for any other purpose without written permission from the copyright owner.

ISBN 0-205-19862-7

Printed in the United States of America

10 9 8 7 6 5 4 3 2 1   01 00 99 98 97 96

Table of Contents

Preface	v
Cross-Reference with Related Texts	vi
World Wide Web Support in the Classroom	xx
List of Transparencies for Exercise Physiology	xxi

CHAPTER 1 The Warm-Up

Outline	1
Suggested Laboratory Activities	3
Review Questions & Answers	4
Exam Questions	10

CHAPTER 2 Respiration

Outline	15
Suggested Laboratory Activities	17
Review Questions & Answers	18
Exam Questions	25

CHAPTER 3 Respiratory Exercise Response, Training Adaptations, And Special Consideration

Outline	31
Suggested Laboratory Activities	33
Review Questions & Answers	34
Exam Questions	40

CHAPTER 4 The Cardiovascular System

Outline	45
Suggested Laboratory Activities	47
Review Questions & Answers	48
Exam Questions	52

CHAPTER 5 Cardiovascular Response To Exercise

Outline	60
Suggested Laboratory Activities	62
Review Questions & Answers	63
Exam Questions	69

CHAPTER 6 Cardiorespiratory Training Principles And Adaptations

Outline	72
Suggested Laboratory Activities	74
Review Questions & Answers	75
Exam Questions	79

CHAPTER 7 Thermoregulation

Outline	83
Suggested Laboratory Activities	85
Review Questions & Answers	86
Exam Questions	90

CHAPTER 8 Cardiorespiratory System Special Applications

Outline	94
Review Questions & Answers	96
Exam Questions	97
Suggested Laboratory Activities	101

CHAPTER 9 Energy Production

Outline	105
Suggested Laboratory Activities	106
Review Questions & Answers	107
Exam Questions	113

CHAPTER 10 Cardiovascular Response To Exercise

Outline	121
Suggested Laboratory Activities	123
Review Questions & Answers	124
Exam Questions	131

CHAPTER 11 Aerobic Metabolism During Exercise

Outline	135
Suggested Laboratory Activities	137
Review Questions & Answers	138
Exam Questions	144

CHAPTER 12 Metabolic Training Principles And Adaptations

Outline	149
Suggested Laboratory Activities	151
Review Questions & Answers	152
Exam Questions	157

CHAPTER 13 Nutrition For Fitness And Athletics

Outline	160
Suggested Laboratory Activities	161
Review Questions & Answers	162
Exam Questions	170

CHAPTER 14 Body Composition: Determination And Importance

Outline	174
Suggested Laboratory Activities	175
Review Questions & Answers	176
Exam Questions	181

CHAPTER 15 Body Composition And Weight Control

Outline	185
Suggested Laboratory Activities	187
Review Questions & Answers	188
Exam Questions	194

CHAPTER 16 Skeletal System

Outline	199
Suggested Laboratory Activities	201
Review Questions & Answers	202
Exam Questions	206

CHAPTER 17 Skeletal Muscle Tissue

Outline	210
Suggested Laboratory Activities	212
Review Questions & Answers	213
Exam Questions	217

CHAPTER 18 Muscular Contraction And Human Movement

Outline	222
Suggested Laboratory Activities	224
Review Questions & Answers	226
Exam Questions	233

CHAPTER 19 Muscular Training Principles And Adaptations

Outline	238
Suggested Laboratory Activities	239
Review Questions & Answers	240
Exam Questions	244

CHAPTER 20 Neuromuscular Aspects Of Movement

Outline	247
Suggested Laboratory Activities	249
Review Questions & Answers	250
Exam Questions	255

PREFACE

This instructor's manual is designed to accompany the textbook ***Exercise Physiology for Health, Fitness and Performance*** by S.A. Plowman and D.L. Smith. Each chapter in this manual corresponds to a chapter in the textbook. Each chapter of the manual contains:

- an expanded outline
- answers for the essay review questions listed at the end of each chapter in the text, along with corresponding page numbers where the answer appears in the text and relevant Figures or Tables that help answer the question.
- suggested laboratory activities
- exam questions (multiple choice and fill in the blank) with answers.

Because of the different way in which this textbook is organized, we have also included a cross-reference table for other frequently used exercise physiology textbooks. This is intended to help faculty members make comparisons and to provide additional reading for students.

Suggestions for how this manual can be made more instructor friendly are solicited from adopters, as well as productive suggestions regarding the text itself.

Cross-Reference of Selected Textbooks with Plowman & Smith

Plowman & Smith	Fox, Bowers & Foss (5th Ed.), 1993	McArdle, Katch, & Katch, 1996
3 units, 20 chapters, 532 pages	6 sections, 22 chapters, 709 pages	2 parts each has 3 sections, 31 chapters, 849 pages

Chapter 1-The Warm-Up
I. What Is Exercise Physiology and Why Study It?
II. Overview of the Text
III. The Exercise Response
  A. Exercise Modalities
  B. Exercise Intensities
  C. Characteristics of the Exerciser
  D. Exercise Task (or Test) Used
  E. Exercise Response Comparisons
IV. Training
  A. Training Adaptations
  B. Training Principles
  C. Health-Related versus Sport-Specific Physical Fitness
  D. Periodization
V. Exercise and Training as Stressors
  A. Selye's Theory of Stress
  B. Physiological Basis of Stress: Neurohormonal Control
  C. Overtraining
	Chapter 1- Introduction to Sports Medicine, Exercise Physiology, and Kinesiology, pgs. 2-9
	Overview of text pgs. 5-8
	
	Chapter 12 pgs. 288-299
		Introduction- Exercise Physiology: Roots and Historical Perspective, pgs. Xiii- xIiii
		
		Chapter 21 pgs. 393-396

Chapter 2- Respiration
I. Introduction
II. Structure of the Pulmonary System
  A. The Conductive Zone
  B. The Respiratory Zone
III. Mechanics of Breathing
IV. Respiratory Circulation
V. Minute Ventilation
VI. Measurement of Lung Volumes
  A. Static Lung Volumes
	Chapter 8 Pulmonary Ventilation pgs. 202-22
	
	pg. 215-216
	pgs. 204-206; rest & exercise
	pgs. 211-213
	pgs. 211-213
		Chapter 12 Pulmonary Structure and Function pgs. 217-232
		
		pgs. 218-222
		
		pgs. 222-225
		pgs. 222-224

B. Dynamic Lung Volumes C. Spirometry D. Gas Dilution E. Standardization	pg. 213	pgs. 224-225
VII. Partial Pressure of a Gas: Dalton's Law	defined Chapter 16, pg. 455, pg. 226	
VIII. Regulation of Pulmonary Ventilation A. The Respiratory Centers B. Anatomical Sensors and Factors Affecting Control of Pulmonary Ventilation	Chapter 11, pg. 269-272	Chapter 13 Gas Exchange and Transport pgs. 235-236; Chapter 14 pgs. 249-263
IX. Gas Exchange and Transport A. Gas Exchange: Henry's Law B. External Respiration C. Internal Respiration D. Oxygen Transport	Chapter 9 pgs. 224-241 Chapter 9 pg.224; Chapter 16 pg. 456 pgs 231-236	chapter 14 pgs. 249-263 pgs. 236-237; 239 pgs. 239-243
X. Arteriovenous Oxygen Difference A. Carbon Dioxide Transport B. The Respiratory System and Acid-Base Balance	pgs. 236-239 Chapter 20 pgs. 578-581	pgs. 244-245 pgs 260-263
Chapter 3- Respiratory Exercise Response, Training Adaptations, And Special Consideration I. Response of the Respiratory System to Exercise A. Short-Term, Submaximal, Light-to Moderate-Intensity Dynamic Aerobic Exercise B. Prolonged, Constant, Relatively Heavy, Submaximal Dynamic Aerobic Exercise C. Incremental Dynamic Aerobic Exercise to Maximum D. Static Exercise E. Entrainment of Respiration During Exercise	Exercise response is in Chapters 8, 9, & 11 ventilation during exercise pgs. 204-205 diffusion capacity during exercise pg. 231 cardiorespiratory control at rest and exercise pg. 273 Material not presented by specific type of exercise	Chapter 14 pgs. 258-260Chapter 12 pgs. 225-231; Chapter 21 pg. 400
II. The Influence of Age and Sex on Respiration at Rest and During Exercise A. Children and Adolescents B. The Elderly C. Male-Female Respiratory Differences	no special section on aging Chapter 14 Exercise Training in Females pg. 368	
III. Respiratory Training Adaptations A. Lung Volumes and Capacities	no special section	Chapter 30 pg. 641

B. Pulmonary Ventilation
C. External and Internal Respiration
D. Why Are There So Few Respiratory Adaptations to Exercise Training?
IV. Special Considerations
   A. The Impact of Altitude on Exercise and Training
   B. Hypoxic Swim Training
   C. Exercise Training and Pollution
	Chapter 16 Diffusion, Osmosis, Scuba, and Performance at Altitude pgs. 461-469
	no special sections
	" "
		Chapter 24 Exercise at Medium and High Altitude pgs. 483-497
		no special sections
		" "

Chapter 4- The Cardiovascular System
I. Introduction
II. Overview of the Cardiovascular System
   A. The Heart
   B. The Vascular System
   C. Blood
   D. Hormonal Control of Blood Volume
III. Cardiovascular Dynamics
   A. Cardiac Output (Q)
   B. Principles of Blood Flow
IV. Regulation of the Cardiovascular System
   A. Neural Control
   B. Anatomical Sensors and Factors Affecting Control of the Cardiovascular System
   C. Neuro-hormonal Control
V. Assessment of Cardiovascular Variables
   A. Cardiac Output
   B. Stroke Volume
   C. Heart Rate
   D. Maximal Oxygen Consumption
   E. Blood Pressure
	Chapter 10 pgs. 242-254
	
	pgs. 244-250
	Chapter 11 pgs. 273-281
	pgs. 255-258
	
	Chapter 11 pgs. 273-281
	no special section
	
	pgs. 258-260
		Chapter 15 The cardiovascular System pgs. 267-283
		
		pgs. 267-268; Chapter 16 pgs. 285-286
		pgs. 268-274
		
		Chapter 16 286-294
		Chapter 17 pgs. 297-298
		
		Chapter 274-278

Chapter 5- Cardiovascular Response To Exercise I. Introduction II. Cardiovascular Responses to Dynamic Aerobic Exercise	Chapter 10 pgs. 250-255, 260-262; Chapter 11 pgs. 274-281	Chapter 7 pgs. 124-126

A. Short Term, Submaximal, Light to Moderate Intensity Exercise B. Prolonged, Heavy, Submaximal Dynamic Exercise C. Incremental Dynamic Exercise to Maximum D. Upper- Body versus Lower-Body Exercise E. Sex Differences During Dynamic Aerobic Exercise F. Responses of Children to Dynamic Aerobic Exercise G. Responses of Elderly to Dynamic Aerobic Exercise III. Cardiovascular Responses to Static Exercise A. Intensity of Muscle Contraction B. Sex Differences in Responses to Static Exercise C. Cardiovascular Response to Static Exercise in Older Adults IV. Cardiovascular Responses to Dynamic Resistance Exercise	Chapter 14 pgs. 387-391 no special section " "	
Chapter 6- Cardiorespiratory Training Principles And Adaptations I. Introduction II. Application of the Training Principles A. Specificity B. Overload C. Individualization D. Adaptation E. Progression F. Maintenance G. Retrogression/Plateau/Reversibility Warm-Up and Cool-Down III. Cardiovascular Adaptations to Endurance Training A. Cardiac Dimensions (1a) B. Coronary Blood Flow (1b)	Chapter 12 pg. 288; Chapter 13 pgs. 345-352; Chapter 15 pgs 429-437 Chapter 13 pgs. 327-343; Chapter 15 pgs. 425-429	Chapter 21 anaerobic changes pgs. 396-398; aerobic changes pgs. 398-401; pgs. 402-412 Chapter 17 pgs. 299-311; Chapter 21 pg. 400

C. Blood Volume (2)		Chapter 17 pgs. 299-300
D. Cardiac Output (3a)		pgs. 300-310
E. Stroke Volume (3b)		
F. Heart Rate (3c)		
G. Maximal Oxygen Consumption (4)		
H. Blood Pressure (5)		
I. Total Peripheral Resistance (6)	Chapter 10 pgs. 255-258	
J. Muscle Blood Flow (7)		
K. Rate-Pressure Product (8)	Chapter 14 pgs. 387-391	
L. Sex Difference in Adaptation		
M. Adaptations in Children		Chapter 30 pgs. 641-643
N. Adaptations in the Elderly		
IV. Cardiovascular Adaptations to Dynamic Resistance Training		
A. Cardiac Dimensions		
B. Stroke Volume and Heart Rate		
C. Blood Pressure		
D. Maximal Oxygen Consumption		Chapter 7 pg. 126
Chapter 7- Thermoregulation	Chapter 17 Heat Balance: Exercise in the Heat and Cold pgs. 472-509	Chapter 25 Exercise and Thermal Stress pgs. 501-525
I. Introduction		
II. Exercise in Environmental Extremes		
III. Basic Concepts		
A. Measurement of Environmental Conditions		
B. Measurement of Body Temperature		
C. Thermal Balance	pg. 475	pgs. 501-502
D. Heat Exchange	pgs. 475-477	pgs. 502-506
E. Heat Exchange During Exercise		
IV. Exercise in the Heat: Cardiovascular Demands	pgs. 481-496	pgs. 507-512
A. Factors Affecting Cardiovascular Response to Exercise in the Heat		
B. Sex Differences in Exercise Response in Heat		pgs. 513-514
C. Exercise Response of Older Adults in the Heat	no special section	
D. Exercise Response of Children in the Heat	" "	pgs. 512-513
E. Heat Illness		pg. 513
V. Exercise in the Cold		

A. Cold-Induced Injuries B. Prevention C. Factors Influencing Cold Tolerance	pgs. 496-505	pgs. 519-522

Chapter 8- Cardiorespiratory System Special Applications
I. Introduction
II. Physical Activity and Cardiovascular Risk Factors
  A. Major Modifiable Risk Factors
  B. Contributing Modifiable Risk Factors
  C. Selected Nontraditional Risk Factors
III. Children and the Cardiovascular Risk Factors
  A. Cholesterol-Lipid Fractions
  B. Cigarette Smoking
  C. Hypertension
  D. Physical Inactivity
  E. Diabetes Mellitus
  F. Obesity
  G. Stress, Fibrinogen, and Fibrinolytic Activity
IV. Immune System, Exercise Training, and Illness
  A. Immune Response
  B. Effect of Exercise on Immune Response
  C. Hormonal Control of Immune Response to Exercise
  D. Training Adaptation
V. Selected Interactions of Exercise and Immune Function
  A. Exercise, the Immune System, and Upper Respiratory Tract Infection
  B. Exercise, the Immune System, and Cancer
  C. Exercise, the Immune System, and Aids
	Chapter 15 exercise Training for Health and Fitness pgs. 412-445
	pgs. 412-425, 437-438
	
	pg. 438
	
	no special section
		Chapter 30 pgs. 645-655
		
		Chapter 20 The Endocrine System pgs. 383-384
		
		Chapter 31 pgs. 673-676

Chapter 9- Energy Production I. Introduction II. Cellular Respiration	Chapter 2 Energy Sources pgs. 13-40	Chapter 5 Introduction to Energy Transfer pgs. 89-99; Chapter 6 Energy Transfer in the Body pgs. 101-119

A. Carbohydrate Metabolism	pgs. 14-25
B. Fat Metabolism	pgs. 25-28
C. Protein Metabolism	pg. 117
III. The Regulation of Cellular Respiration and ATP Production	
A. Intracellular	
B. Extracellular	
C. Neurohormonal Coordination	Chapter 21 pgs. 30-37
IV. Fuel Utilization at Rest and During Exercise	Chapter 9 pgs. 151-158
Chapter 10- Cardiovascular Response To Exercise	
I. The Energy Continuum	pg. 37
II. Measurement of Anaerobic Metabolism	Chapter 4 pgs. 64-68
A. Laboratory Procedures	
III. The Anaerobic Exercise Response	
A. Oxygen Deficit and Excess Postexercise Oxygen Consumption	Chapter 2 pgs. 33-37; Chapter 3 pgs. 44-53
B. ATP-PC Changes	
C. Lactate Changes	Chapter 3 pgs. 53-57
IV. Male vs. Female Anaerobic Characteristics	Chapter 14 pgs. 44-53
A. The Availability and Utilization of ATP-PC	
B. The Accumulation of Lactate	
C. Mechanical Power and Capacity	
V. Anaerobic Exercise Characteristics of Children	Chapter 11 pg. 194
A. The Availability and Utilization of ATP-PC	
B. The Accumulation of Lactate	
C. The Lactate Threshold(s)	
D. Mechanical Power and Capacity	
VI. Anaerobic Exercise Characteristics of Older Adults	
A. The Availability and Utilization of ATP-PC	
B. The Accumulation of Lactate	
C. Mechanical Power and Capacity	
VII. Heritability of Anaerobic Characteristics	

pgs. 108-115
pgs. 115-117
pg. 117

Chapter 9 pgs. 151-158

Chapter 7 pgs. 121-137
Chapter 7 pgs. 129-130
Chapter 11 pgs. 191-194

Chapter 7 pgs. 130-135

Chapter 11 pgs. 191-196

Chapter 11- Aerobic Metabolism During Exercise
I. Introduction
II. Laboratory Measurement of Aerobic Metabolism
   A. Calorimetry
   B. Spirometry
III. Aerobic Exercise Responses
   A. Oxygen Consumption and Carbon Dioxide Production
   B. The Oxygen Cost of Breathing
   C. Respiratory Quotient/Respiratory Exchange Ratio
   D. Lactate Changes
   E. Estimation of Caloric Intake and Expenditure
   F. The Metabolic Equivalent (MET)
IV. Field Estimates of Energy Expenditure During Exercise
   A. Metabolic Calculations Based on Mechanical Work or Standard Energy Use
   B. Motion Sensors and Accelerometers
   C. Activity Recalls and Questionnaires
V. Efficiency and Economy
   A. Efficiency
   B. Economy of Walking and Running
VI. Why Do Economy and Efficiency Matter?
VII. Heritability of Aerobic Characteristics
	Chapter 13 pgs. 352-354
	
	Chapter 4 pgs. 64-68, 77-78
	
	Chapter 4 pgs. 68-73
	
	pgs. 70-73
	
	pgs 78-79
	pgs. 84-87
	
	pgs. 87-89
	
	Chapter 4 pgs. 79-84
		Chapter 4 Energy Value of Food pgs. 83-87; Chapter 8 Measurement of Human energy Expenditure pgs. 139-149
		
		Chapter 4 pgs. 83-84; Chapter 8 pgs. 139-140
		Chapter 8 pgs. 140-145; Chapter 11 pgs. 200-202
		
		Chapter 8 pgs. 145-148
		
		Chapter 9 pg. 159
		Chapter 9 pgs. 161-162; Chapter 11 pgs. 207-210
		
		Chapter 10 pgs. 167-184

Chapter 12- Metabolic Training Principles And Adaptations
I. Introduction
II. Application of the Training Principles for Metabolic Enhancement
   A. Specificity
   B. Overload
	Chapter 12 pg. 286; Chapter 13 pg. 322	

C. Adaptation		
D. Progression		
E. Individualization		
F. Maintenance		
G. Retrogression/Plateau/Reversibility		
H. Warm-Up and Cool-Down		Chapter 11 pgs. 197-200; Chapter 21 pgs. 399-400
III. Metabolic Adaptations to Exercise Training		
A. Substrate or Fuel Supply		
B. Enzyme Activity		
C. Oxygen Utilization		Chapter 7 pgs. 130-135
D. Lactate Accumulation		
E. ATP Production, Storage, and Turnover		
IV. The Influence of Age and Sex on Metabolic Training Adaptations	Chapter 14 pgs. 375-380	
V. The Impact of Genetics on Metabolic Trainability	Chapter 13 pgs. 352-354	Chapter 11 pgs. 203-204
A. Submaximal Substrate or Fuel Utilization		
B. Maximal Work Output and Oxygen Consumption		
C. Genetic Variability		
Chapter 13- Nutrition For Fitness And Athletics	Chapter 18 pgs. 513-536	Chapter 1 Carbohydrates, Lipids, and Protein pgs. 5-53; Chapter 2 Vitamins, Mineral, and Water pgs. 36-59; Chapter 3 Optimal Nutrition for Exercise
I. Introduction		pgs. 61-87
II. Nutrition and Training		
A. Kilocalories	pgs. 514-515	pgs. 5-12
B. Carbohydrate	pgs. 516-519	pgs. 24-28
C. Protein	pgs. 515-516	pgs. 15-22
D. Fat	pgs. 519-521	pgs. 35-42
E. Vitamins	" "	pgs. 42-53
F. Minerals	Chapter 18 pg. 52	
III. Nutrition for Competition		
A. Carbohydrate Loading (Glycogen Supercompensation)	pgs. 528-530	pgs. 12-15; 22-23; 28-31
B. Pre-event Meal	pgs. 524-526	pgs. 72-73
C. Feeding During Exercise	pgs. 526-527	pg. 72
D. Fluid Ingestion During and After Exercise	pg. 527	pgs. 73-74
IV. Eating Disorders	no special section	Chapter 27 pgs. 56-569

Chapter 14- Body Composition: Determination And Importance
 	
I. Introduction
II. Body Composition Assessment
  A. Laboratory Techniques
  B. Field Tests of Body Composition
III. Overweight and Obesity
  A. What Happens to Adipose Cells in Obesity?
    The Cellular Basis of Obesity
  B. Fat Distribution Patterns
  C. Waist-to-Hip Ratio
  D. Health Risks of Overweight and Obesity
IV. Heredity and Body Composition
	Chapter 19 Exercise, Body Composition and Weight Control pgs. 538-574
	
	pgs. 545-551
	
	Chapter 19 pgs. 551-552
		Chapter 27 Body Composition Assessment pgs. 541-575
		
		pgs. 541-569
		
		Chapter 29 Obesity and Weight Control pgs. 603-633; Chapter 30 pgs. 643-644 aging
		
		pg. 609

Chapter 15- Body Composition And Weight Control
 	
I. The Caloric Balance Equation
  A. Food Ingested
  B. Resting or Basal Metabolism
  C. Thermogenesis
  D. The Impact of Diet, Exercise and Exercise Training on Energy Expenditure
  E. The Effect of Diet, Exercise Training, and Diet Plus Exercise Training on Body Composition and Weight
II. Applications of the Training Principles for Weight and Body Composition Loss and/or Control
  A. Specificity
  B. Overload
  C. Adaptation
  D. Progression
  E. Individualization
  F. Retrogression/Plateau/Reversibility
  G. Maintenance
III. Making Weight for Sport
	Chapter 19 pgs. 553-565
	
	Chapter 19 pgs. 566-568
		Chapter 28 pgs. 595-599; chapter 29 pgs. 616-628
		
		Chapter 28 Physique, Performance, and Physical Activity pgs. 577-595

Chapter 16- Skeletal System
I. Introduction
II. Skeletal Tissue
   A. Functions
   B. Levels of Organization
   C. Bone Development
III. Assessment of Bone Health
   A. Laboratory Measures
   B. Field Tests
IV. Factors Influencing Bone Health
   A. Age-related Changes in Bone
   B. Sex Differences in Bone Mineral Density
   C. Development of Peak Bone Mass
V. Exercise Response
VI. Application of the Training Principles
   A. Specificity
   B. Overload
   C. Individualization
   D. Retrogression/Plateau
   E. Warm-up/Cool-down
VII. Skeletal Adaptations to Exercise Training
VII. Special Applications to Health and Fitness Function, and Bone Density
   A. Osteoporosis
   B. Physical Activity, Altered Menstrual
   C. Skeletal Injuries
	No similar chapter
	
	Chapter 14
	
	Chapter 14
		Chapter 27 pgs. 566-569
		
		Chapter 2 pgs. 45-47
		
		Chapter 22 pgs. 446-447, 1 section on muscle strength and BMD
		Chapter 30 pgs. 644-645
		
		Chapter 2 pgs. 45-47

Chapter 17- Skeletal Muscle Tissue
I. Introduction
II. Overview of Muscle Tissue
   A. Functions of Skeletal Muscle
   B. Characteristics of Muscle Tissue
III. Macroscopic Structure of Skeletal Muscles
   A. Organization and Connective Tissue
   B. Architectural Organization
	Chapter 5 Skeletal Muscle: Structure and Function pgs. 94-135
	
	pgs. 96-98
		Chapter 18 Skeletal Muscle: Structure and Function pgs. 315-336
		
		pgs. 315-317

IV. Microscopic Structure of a Muscle Fiber
    A. Muscle Fibers
V. Molecular Structure of the Myofilaments
    A. Thick Filaments
    B. Thin Filaments
VI. Contraction of a Muscle Fiber
    A. The Sliding Filament Theory of Muscle Contraction
    B. Excitation-Contraction Coupling
    C. Changes in the Sarcomere During Contraction
    D. All-or-none Principle
VII. Muscle Fiber Types
    A. Assessment of Muscle Fiber Type
    B. Distribution of Fiber Types
    C. Fiber Type in Athletes
	pgs. 98-99
	
	pgs. 99-101
	
	pgs. 101-107
	
	pgs. 107-129
	pgs. 110-113
	pgs. 120-122
		pgs. 317-318
		
		pgs. 321-324
		
		pgs. 324-328
		
		pgs. 328-330
		
		pgs. 330-334

Chapter 18- Muscular Contraction And Human Movement
I. Exercise - The Result of Muscle Contraction
    A. Tension versus Load
    B. Classification of Muscle Contractions
    C. Force Development or Variation and Gradation of Response
    D. Muscular Fatigue and Soreness
II. Assessing Muscular Function
    A. Laboratory Methods
    B. Laboratory and Field Methods
    C. Field Tests
III. Age, Sex and Muscle Function
IV. Heritability of Muscular Function
	Chapter 5 pgs. 122-124; Chapter 7 pgs. 160-166
	
	Chapter 5 124-129; Chapter 7 pgs. 172-174
	Chapter 7 pgs. 163-166
	
	Chapter 14 pgs. 380-387
		Chapter 22 pgs. 448-451
		pgs. 417-420
		pgs. 430-439
		
		pgs. 421-426; pg. 427; Chapter 30 pgs. 639-641

Chapter 19- Muscular Training Principles And Adaptations	Chapter 7 Development of Muscular Strength, Endurance, and Flexibility pgs. 158-199	Chapter 22 Muscular strength: Training Muscles to Become Stronger pgs. 417-455

I. Introduction
II. Muscular Training
  A. Overview of Resistance Training
III. Application of the Training Principles
  A. Specificity
  B. Overload
  C. Adaptation
  D. Progression
  E. Individualization
  F. Maintenance
  G. Retrogression/Plateau/Reversibility
  H. Warm-Up and Cool Down
  I. Specific Application of Training Principles to Body Building
IV. Muscular Adaptations to Exercise Training
  A. Neuromuscular Adaptations to Resistance Training Programs
  B. Muscle Adaptations to Endurance Training Programs
V. Special Applications
  A. Muscular Strength and Endurance and Lower-Back Pain
  B. Anabolic Steroids
	pgs. 175-185
	pgs. 170-172
	
	Chapter 7 pgs. 166-170
	
	Chapter 22 pgs. 617-621
		pgs. 426-429; pgs. 440-448
		
		Chapter 22 pgs. 429-430

Chapter 20- Neuromuscular Aspects Of Movement
I. Introduction
II. Neural Control of Muscle Fibers
  A. Nerve Supply
  B. The Neuromuscular Junction
III. Reflex Control of Movement
  A. Spinal Cord
  B. Components of a Reflex Arc
  C. Proprioceptors and Reflexes
IV. Volitional Control of Movement
  A. Volitional Control of Individual Motor Units
  B. Volitional Control of Muscle Movement
	Chapter 6 Nervous control of Muscular Movement pgs. 136-157
	pgs. 138-145
		Chapter 23 pgs. 457-460
		Chapter 19 Neural Control of Human Movement pgs. 339-355

V. Flexibility
    A. Assessing Flexibility   Chapter 7 pgs. 185-193
    B. The Influence of Age and Sex on Flexibility   pgs. 186-187
    C. Flexibility and Low-Back Pain
    D. Flexibility Training
VI. Application of the Training Principles
    A. Specificity   pgs. 187-190
    B. Overload   Chapter 7 pgs. 187-192
    C. Adaptation and Progression
    D. Individualization
    E. Maintenance
    F. Retrogression/Plateau/Reversibility
    G. Warm-Up and Cool-Down
VII. Adaptation to Flexibility Training

World Wide Web Support in the Classroom
Suggested Activities

The Internet is becoming a useful tool in many educational settings, including the teaching of Exercise Physiology. Recognizing the increased reliance on the World Wide Web to support classroom activities and academic projects, we are including some WWW addresses that we have found useful. Additionally, you and your students may want to visit the Website for the textbook, which can be accessed through the Allyn & Bacon Homepage (WWW.abacon.com).

Health and Fitness Links
http://pc-33.kines.uiuc.edu/links/health.html

Kinesiology/Physical Education Departments with Homepages
http://www/niu.edu/acad/phed/homepage.html
http://pc-33.kines.uiuc.edu/links/depts.html
http://www/angelfire.com/pages0/jdemmett/index.html
http://www.louisville.edu/~pcmyerz1
http://yoda.ucc.uconn.edu.yiannakisa.Gradguid.html
http://rohan.sdsu.edu/dept/spincarl/fradstud.html
see links at http://garnet.berkeley.edu/~hbbiomxl/dferris.useful.html (extensive list)

Organizations
American Alliance for Health, Physical Education, Recreation and Dance (AAHPERD)
        http://www.aahperd.org
American College of Sports Medicine (ACSM)   http://www.acsm.org
Gatorade Sports and Science Institute (GSSI)   http://www.gssiweb.com
Related Organizations (list)
        http://www.loisville.edu~pcmyerz1/areas/areas.html
see links at http://garnet.berkeley.edu/~hbbiomxl/dferris.useful.html

Research Funding Agencies
http://www.cs.virgina.edu/˜resdev/sponsors.html
see links at http://garnet.berkeley.edu/~hbbiomxl/dferris.useful.html

Resources
http://www.uiuc.edu/ref/research.html
http://www.gen.emory.edu/medweb/medweb.physiology.html
http://www.netrunner.net/~irssurf
see links at http://garnet.berkeley.edu/~hbbiomxl/dferris.useful.html

As always, we welcome your suggestions regarding additional Websites that you believe should be added to this list.

Transparencies for Exercise Physiology

Figure 1.1	Schematic Representation of Text Organization
Figure 1.2	The Comparative Basis for Exercise Responses and Training Adaptations
Figure 1.4	Physical Fitness
Figure 1.5	Periodization for Training Athletes
Figure 1.6	Pathways of Neurohormonal Regulation of the Exercise Stress Response
Figure 2.8	Factors that Influence the Control of Pulmonary Ventilation
Figure 2.11	Oxygen and Carbon Dioxide Exchange
Figure 2.13	Oxygen Dissociation Curve
Figure 2.14	Summary of Oxygen and Carbon Dioxide Transport
Figure 3.1	Responses of Pulmonary Ventilation Variables to Constant, Submaximal Dynamic Exercise
Figure 3.2	Responses of External Respiration Variables to Constant, Submaximal Dynamic Exercise
Figure 3.3	Oxygen Dissociation During Exercise
Figure 3.5	Responses of Internal Respiration Variables to Constant, Submaximal Dynamic Exercise
Figure 3.7	Responses of External Respiration Variables to Prolonged, Constant, Submaximal Dynamic Exercise
Figure 3.8	Responses of Internal Respiration Variables to Prolonged, Constant, Submaximal Dynamic Exercise
Figure 3.9	Responses of Pulmonary Ventilation Variables to Incremental Dynamic Exercise to Maximum
Figure 3.10	Responses of External Respiration Variables to Incremental Dynamic Exercise to Maximum
Figure 3.11	Responses of Internal Respiration Variables to Incremental Dynamic Exercise to Maximum
Figure 4.3	Conduction System of the Heart
Figure 4.4	Periods of the Cardiac Cycle
Figure 4.5	Summary of the Cardiac Cycle
Figure 4.12	Relationships among CSA of Blood vessels, Blood Pressure and Resistance
Figure 4.14	Factors Affecting Neural Control of the Cardiovascular System
Figure 5.1	Cardiovascular Responses to Short-term, Light to Moderate, Dynamic Exercise
Figure 5.4	Cardiovascular Responses to Prolonged, Heavy, Dynamic Exercise
Figure 5.5	Cardiovascular Responses to Prolonged, Heavy, Dynamic Exercise with and without Fluid Replacement
Figure 5.7	Cardiovascular Responses to Incremental, Dynamic Exercise

Figure 5.10	Cardiovascular Responses to Incremental, Dynamic Exercise Upper-Body and Lower-Body Exercises
Figure 5.11	Comparison of Cardiovascular Responses of Men and Women to Submaximal Exercise
Figure 5.15	Maximal Oxygen Consumption and Endurance Performance in Children and Adolescents
Figure 5.17	Cardiovascular Responses to Varying Intensities of Forearm Contraction
Figure 5.18	Blood Flow in the Quadriceps Muscle During Different Intensities of Contraction
Figure 5.19	Comparison of Heart Rate and Blood Pressure Responses to Static and Dynamic Exercise
Figure 5.23	Heart Rate and Blood Pressure Response to Resistance Exercise
Figure 6.1	Changes in VO2max Based on Frequency, Intensity, and Duration of Training and on Initial Fitness Level
Figure 6.3	Effects of Reducing Exercise Frequency, Intensity, and Duration on Maintenance of VO2max
Figure 6.5	Sites of Cardiovascular Adaptations to Dynamic Endurance Training
Figure 6.6	Changes in Blood Volume as a Result of Training and Detraining
Figure 6.7	Comparison of Cardiovascular Response of Trained and Untrained Individuals to Incremental Exercise to Maximum
Figure 7.6	Cardiovascular Responses to Hot or Thermoneutral Conditions
Figure 7.8	Comparisons of Rectal Temperature, Heart Rate, and Sweat Loss in Acclimated and Unacclimated Individuals during Prolonged Exercise
Figure 8.3	Overview of Immune System
Figure 8.5	The "Open-Window" Hypothesis
Figure 9.2	An Overview of Cellular Respiration
Figure 9.5	Glycolysis
Figure 9.7	Stage II: The Formation of Acetyl CoA
Figure 9.8	Stage III: The Krebs Cycle
Figure 9.9	Stage IV: Electron Transport and Oxidative Phosphorylation
Figure 9.11	Cellular Respiration
Figure 9.16	Extracellular Neurohormonal Regulation of Metabolism
Figure 10.1	Anaerobic and Aerobic Sources of ATP
Figure 10.2	Time-Energy System Continuum
Figure 10.5	Oxygen Deficit and EPOC during Submaximal Exercise and Supramaximal Exercise
Figure 10.7	Time Course for the Depletion of CP and ATP and the Accumulation of Lactate as a Consequence of Incremental Exercise
Figure 10.9	Ventilatory and Lactate Thresholds During Incremental Work to Maximum

Figure 10.10	The Rate of Appearance, the Rate of Disappearance and the Resultant Accumulation of Lactate as a Consequence of Incremental Exercise
Figure 10.11	The Time Course of Lactate Removal during Resting Recovery from Exercise
Figure 10.14	Lactate Values After Maximal Exercise as a Function of Age and Sex
Figure 11.4	Oxygen Consumption Responses to Various Exercises
Figure 11.5	Respiratory and Metabolic Responses to Heavy Static Exercise
Figure 11.6	Lactate Accumulation during Short- and Long-Term Constant Submaximal Exercise
Figure 11.8	Lactate Accumulation Resulting from Increasing Distance of Competitive Running Races
Figure 11.13	The Economy of Walking and Running for Children vs. Adults
Figure 11.17	Predicted Velocity of VO2max
Figure 12.1	Metabolic Training Adaptations
Figure 13.4	Nutrient Intake in Elite Norwegian Female Athletes
Figure 14.3	Estimated Changes in Fat Free Body Composition as a Function of Age
Figure 14.7	Percent Body Fat Changes with Age
Figure 15.1	Energy Expenditure
Figure 15.3	Effects of Diet, Exercise, Training, and Diet Plus Exercise on the Composition of Weight Loss
Figure 15.6	Importance of Exercise in Maintaining Weight Loss
Figure 16.2	Stages of Bone Remodeling
Figure 16.7	Bone Density Comparison
Figure 17.2	Organization of Skeletal Tissue
Figure 17.4	Organization of a Muscle Fiber
Figure 17.9	Regulatory Function of Troponin and Tropomyosin
Figure 17.10	Phases of Excitation Contraction Coupling
Figure 17.11	Force Generation of the Contractile Elements: The Cross-bridging Cycle
Figure 17.13	Properties of Motor Units
Figure 17.15	Force Production and Fatigue Curves of Fiber Types
Figure 18.2	Length-Tension Relationship in Skeletal Muscle Fibers
Figure 18.5	Strength Curves for Knee Flexion
Figure 18.6	Strength Curves for Hip Abduction
Figure 18.7	Strength Curves for Elbow Flexion
Figure 18.8	Strength Curves for Knee Extension
Figure 18.10	Force-Velocity Curves
Figure 18.11	Influence of Fiber Type on Velocity

Figure 18.14	Possible Sites of Muscle Fatigue
Figure 18.15	An Integrated Model to Explain DOMS
Figure 18.18	Strength Development in Boys and Girls
Figure 18.22	Growth Curves for Mass and Percent Fat in Children
Figure 18.24	Loss of Muscle Fibers with Age
Figure 19.1	Theoretical Continuum Presenting Characteristics of a Training Program
Figure 19.3	Neuromuscular Adaptations to a Resistance Training Program
Figure 20.5	Components of a Reflex Arc
Figure 20.6	Neuromuscular Spindle
Figure 20.7	Myotatic Reflex
Figure 20.9	Inverse Myotatic Reflex
Figure 20.13	Flexibility in Males and Females

Chapter 1

THE WARM-UP

Outline

I. What Is Exercise Physiology and Why Study It?

II. Overview of the Text

III. The Exercise Response

    A. Exercise Modalities

    B. Exercise Intensities

    C. Characteristics of the Exerciser

    D. Exercise Task (or Test) Used

    E. Exercise Response Comparisons

IV. Training

    A. Training Adaptations

    B. Training Principles

        1. Specificity

        2. Overload

        3. Adaptation

        4. Progression

        5. Retrogression/Plateau/Reversibility

        6. Maintenance

        7. Individualization

        8. Warm-Up/Cool-Down

    C. Health-Related versus Sport-Specific Physical Fitness

D. Periodization

V. Exercise and Training as Stressors

   A. Selye's Theory of Stress

   B. Physiological Basis of Stress: Neurohormonal Control

   C. Overtraining

THE WARM-UP

Suggested Laboratory Activities

1. Have students take a variety of physical fitness tests. Identify each as a Health-related or Sport-specific physical fitness test.

2. Present a training program. Have students identify how each training principle is incorporated into this program.

3. Present a series of work-outs in randomized order for a selected sport. Have students arrange these in the periodization macrocycles: rest; off-season; pre-season; in-season (early or late).

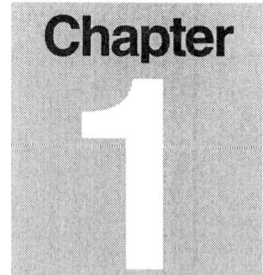

THE WARM UP
Review Questions

1. Define *exercise physiology, exercise* and *exercise training*.

   Pg. 2
   Exercise physiology is both a basic and an applied science that describes, explains, and uses the body's response to exercise and adaptation to exercise training to maximize human physical potential.

   Pg. 5
   Exercise is a single bout of bodily exertion or muscular activity that requires an expenditure of energy above resting level and results in voluntary movement.

   Pg. 8
   Exercise training is a consistent or chronic progression of exercise sessions designed to improve physiological function for better health or sport performance.

2. Explain the comparisons used to describe the exercise response and training adaptations.

   Figure 1.2; Pgs. 7-8
   Submaximal and maximal exercise responses are compared to resting values for any variable. Post training levels of any variable are compared to pretraining levels of the same condition: T_2 rest vs. T_1 rest; T_2 submax vs. T_1 submax; T_2 max vs. T_1 max

3. Differentiate between an absolute and relative submaximal workload, and give an example using a situation other than weight lifting.

   Pg. 6
   During submaximal exercise the workload may be described in two ways, as an absolute workload or a relative workload. An absolute submaximal workload is one that is known or assumed to be below

an individual's maximum and is constant for everyone. This workload does not take into account individual differences in fitness levels. An example would be to have all class members exercise at 150 b·min^{-1}. This may be a very light workload for some and a very high workload for others. Conversely, a relative submaximal workload individualizes a workload for each person. A relative heart rate workload may be to ask each person to work at a heart rate of 60% of heart rate max. This may be 96 b·min^{-1} for an older individual and 120 b·min^{-1} for a younger individual.

4. Fully describe an exercise situation, including all elements that are needed to accurately evaluate the exercise response.

> **Pgs. 5-7**
> To describe an exercise response four factors must be considered; the *exercise modality*, the *exercise intensity*, the *characteristics of the exerciser*, and the *exercise task*. In describing the exercise response to a 3 mile run in a 30 year old male ex-cross country runner:
> A) *Exercise modality*- the modality is running
> B) *Exercise intensity*- the intensity will be assessed or monitored by the heart rate response during an 18 minute, 3 mile run.
> C) *Characteristics of the exerciser* - the ability of the exerciser will influence the exercise response. Since the exerciser can run 3 miles in 18 minutes, it is apparent that this exerciser has running abilities above the normal 30 year old male.
> D) *Exercise task* -the exercise task is the 3 mile run in 18 minutes.

5. Differentiate between the three levels of training adaptation, and state which level of adaptation is most common.

> **Pgs. 8-9**
> The three levels of training adaptation are chronic change, last-bout effect, and augmented last-bout effect. A chronic change is an adaptation that occurs as the result of training and will remain as long as the training continues. A last-bout effect is a temporary positive change that lasts only a matter of hours after the exercise session. The augmented last-bout occurs when the positive, but still temporary post-exercise change increases over a period of one to several weeks until a limit is reached.. The chronic change is the adaptation the is most common.

6. List and explain the training principals.

Pgs. 9-10
- *Specificity*- The body will adapt to the specific demands placed upon it; training programs must match goals.
- *Overload*- To place a demand on the body that is greater than it is accustomed to. Three factors must be considered, the intensity of the exercise, the duration of the exercise, and the frequency of the exercise.
- *Adaptation*- The change in physiological function that occurs in response to training.
- *Progression*- The change in overload in response to adaptation.
- *Retrogression/Plateau/Reversibility*- Describes possible rate of change that may occur with training. When performances plateau or get worse it may be the signs of overtraining. When training stops, detraining or a reversal of adaptations may occur.
- *Maintenance*- The sustaining of an achieved adaptation.
- *Individualization*- The individual rate of response that will occur from a training program. The necessity of prescribing exercise to match the goals and abilities of each individual.
- *Warm-Up/ Cool-Down*- Preparing the body for activity by elevating body temperature/ slowly bringing the body temperature back to pre-exercise levels.

7. Compare the components of health-related physical fitness with those of sport-specific physical fitness.

Figure 1.4; Pgs. 10-11
Health-related physical fitness is the portion of physical fitness which is directed toward the prevention of or rehabilitation from disease. Sport-specific physical fitness is that portion of physical fitness directed toward optimizing athletic performance. Health-related physical fitness components include cardiovascular-respiratory endurance, body composition, and muscular fitness (strength, endurance and flexibility). Sport-specific physical fitness components include those of health-related physical fitness and add to this list other components specific to the particular sport (agility, balance [static and dynamic], power and/or anaerobic power and capacity.

8. Diagram and give an example of periodization for a sport of your choice.

Figure 1.5; Pgs. 11-13

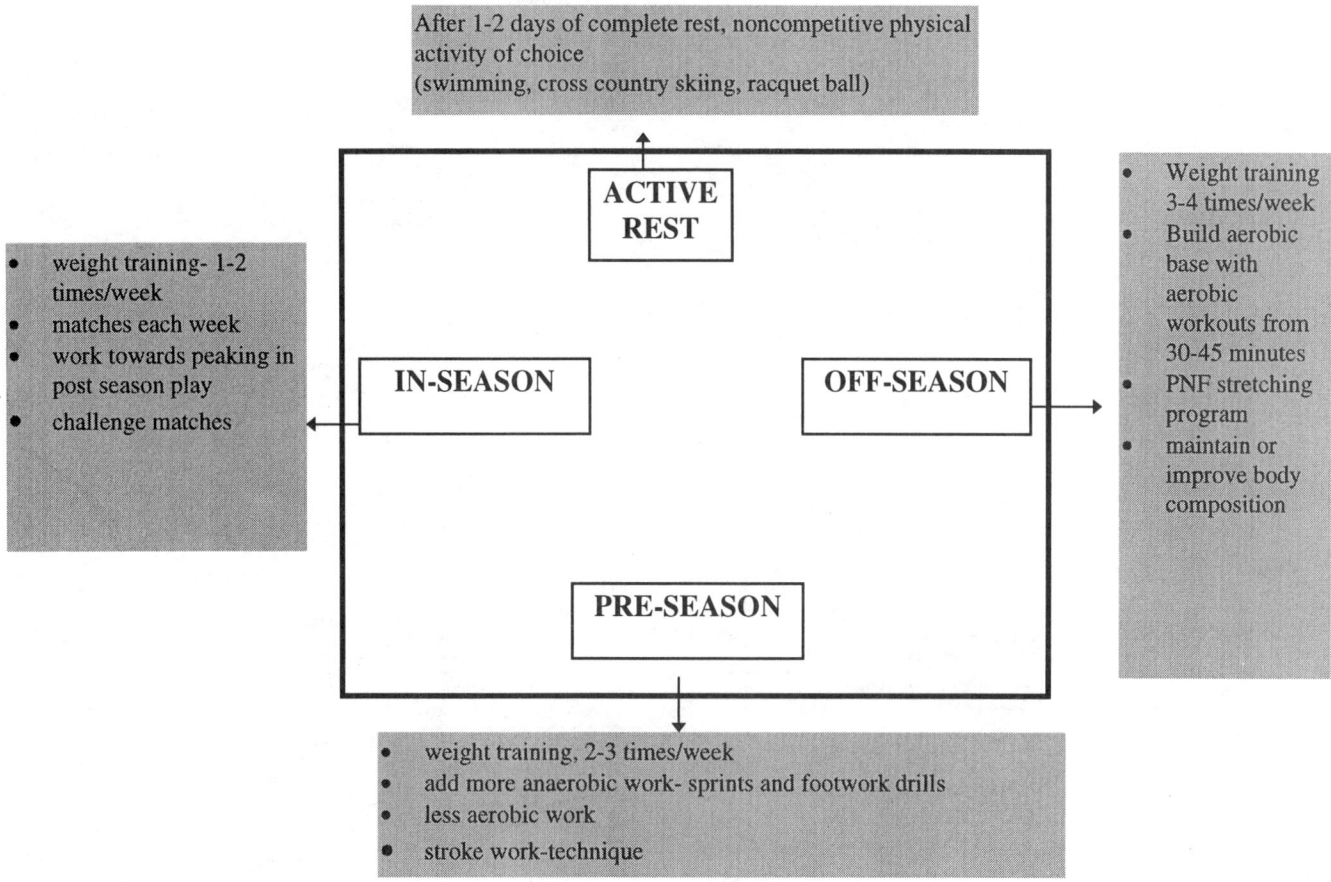

9. Prepare a line chart of the neurohormonal physiological basis of the exercise and exercise training stress response.

Figure 1.6; Pgs. 13-14

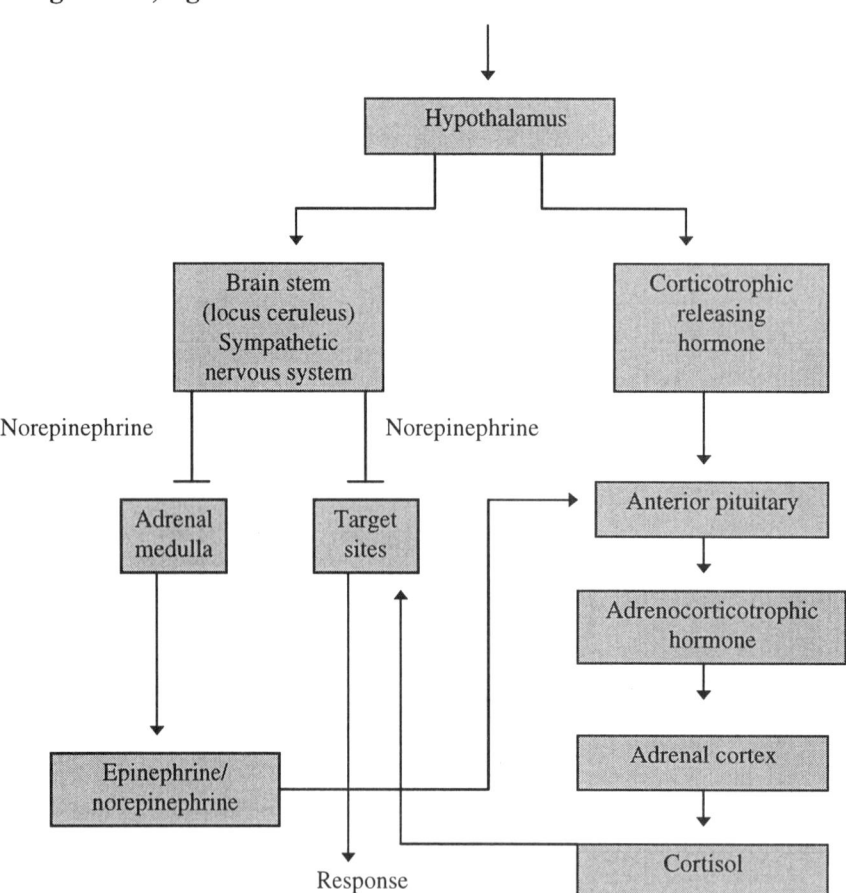

10. Identify the performance-related, physiological, and behavioral signs and symptoms of overtraining that can be evaluated with little if any laboratory testing.

Table 1.1, Pg. 15

Performance-Related	Physiological	Behavioral
<ul><li>consistent decrement in performance</li><li>persistent fatigue and sluggishness that leads to poor training sessions</li><li>prolonged recovery from training</li><li>reappearance of already corrected skills</li></ul>	<ul><li>decreased maximal work capacities</li><li>headaches or stomachaches</li><li>insomnia</li><li>persistent low-grade stiffness and soreness</li><li>frequent sore throats, colds or cold sores</li><li>loss of appetite, body weight</li><li>elevation of morning heart rate</li></ul>	<ul><li>feelings of depression</li><li>general apathy</li><li>difficulty concentrating</li><li>loss of competitive drive</li></ul>

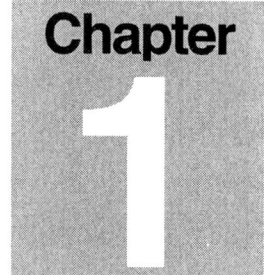

THE WARM-UP
Exam Questions

A. Multiple Choice

1. Overtraining is an indication that the individual is not physiologically adapting to the stress of exercise training, probably because of:
   a. psychological pressures associated with performance.
   b. large, abrupt increases in training load.
   c. insufficient attention being paid to rest and recovery.
   d. a, b, and c are correct
   e. b and c are correct

   Answer- e

2. The majority of the adaptations which occur as a result of exercise training may be described as:
   a. a last bout effect.
   b. an augmented last bout effect.
   c. a chronic change.
   d. an acute response.

   Answer- c

3. The test utilized to evoke an exercise response needs to be taken into account when interpreting the results.
   a. Criterion tests and field tests are generally of equal accuracy.
   b. All laboratory tests are criterion tests.
   c. Field tests are often performance based and often estimate values measured by the criterion test.
   d. Field tests should always be selected even if a criterion test is easily available, since the general public understands them easier.

   Answer- c

4. The primary exercise modalities can be described by energy production type or muscle action. Which categories are appropriate if the description is by muscle action for exercise physiology?
   a. agonists and antagonists
   b. aerobic and anaerobic
   c. continuous rhythmical endurance, dynamic resistance, and static
   d. submaximal short light intensity, submaximal long, heavy intensity, maximal

Answer- c

5. Which of the following describes an exercise task in which the individual is most likely to achieve a steady state and maintain it for the duration?
   a. submaximal, short, light to moderate intensity exercise
   b. submaximal, long, moderate to heavy intensity exercise
   c. incremental work to maximum
   d. dynamic resistance activity

Answer- a

6. When describing the physiological exercise response, it is important to:
   a. establish whether the exercise modality is aerobic endurance or anaerobic resistance.
   b. use the individual's maximal capacity as the baseline for comparison.
   c. describe whether the exercise intensity is maximal or submaximal.
   d. all of the above
   e. a and c

Answer- e

7. In describing the physiologic adaptation to exercise training:
   a. The baseline for comparison is the same condition (rest, submaximal or maximal exercise) before training.
   b. Most, but not all, variables will increase at maximum.
   c. Most, but not all, variables will increase at rest.
   d. all of the above
   e. a and b

Answer- e

8. Hypokinetic disease:
   a. is caused by a lack of physical activity.
   b. can affect anyone regardless of age or sex.
   c. can lead to serious illnesses.
   d. all of the above

Answer- d

9. The order of the three stages of the General Adaptation Syndrome are:
   1. Resistance   2. Exhaustion   3. Alarm Reaction
   a. 3, 1, 2
   b. 1, 2, 3
   c. 2, 3, 1
   d. 1, 3, 2

Answer- a

10. Periodization is:
    a. when a female begins to menstruate.
    b. a timeline for training cycles.
    c. adjusting to training during the shorter daylight months of the winter.
    d. allowing a sufficient period of time for full recovery from training.

Answer- b

B. Fill in the Blank

1. _____ _____ is a basic and an applied science that describes, explains, and uses the body's response to exercise and adaptation to exercise training to maximize human physical potential.
   Answer- Exercise Physiology

2. _____ is a single acute bout of bodily exertion or muscular activity that requires an expenditure of energy above resting level and that in most, but not all, cases results in voluntary movement.
   Answer- Exercise

3. _____ _____ is the type of activity or sport; usually classified by energy demand or type of muscle action.
   Answer- Exercise Modality or Mode

4. The highest intensity, greatest load, or longest duration exercise of which an individual is capable is called _____ _____.
   Answer- Maximal Exercise

5. A set exercise load performed at any intensity from just above resting to just below maximum is called _____ _____.
   Answer- Absolute Submaximal Workload

6. A workload above resting but below maximum that is prorated to each individual; typically set as some percentage of maximum is called _____ _____.
   Answer- Relative Submaximal Workload

7. _____ _____ is the standard against which other tests are judged.
   Answer- Criterion Test

8. _____ _____ is the precise direct measurement of physiological functions for the assessment of exercise responses or training adaptations; usually involves monitoring, collection, and analysis of expired air, blood, or electrical signals.
Answer- Laboratory Test

9. _____ _____ is a test that can be conducted anywhere; is performance-based and estimates the values measured by the criterion test.
Answer- Field Test

10. A consistent or chronic progression of exercise sessions designed to improve physiological function for better health or sport performance is called _____.
Answer- Training

11. Physiological changes or adjustments resulting from an exercise training program that promote optimal functioning are called _____ _____.
Answer- Training Adaptations

12. Fundamental guidelines that form the basis for the development of an exercise training program are called _____ _____.
Answer- Training Principles

13. _____ _____ is that portion of physical fitness directed toward the prevention of or rehabilitation from disease as well as the development of a high level of functional capacity for the necessary and discretionary tasks of life.
Answer- Health-Related Physical Fitness

14. _____ _____ are diseases caused by and/or associated with lack of physical activity.
Answer- Hypokinetic Diseases

15. That portion of physical fitness which is directed toward optimizing athletic performance is called _____ _____.
Answer- Sport-Specific Physical Fitness

16. A physiological state of well being that provides the foundation for the tasks of daily living, a degree of protection against hypokinetic disease, and a basis for participation in sport is called _____ _____.
Answer- Physical Fitness

17. Plans for training based on a manipulation of the fitness components with the intent of peaking the athlete for the competitive season or varying health-related fitness training in cycles of harder or easier training is called _____ _____.
Answer- Periodization

18. _____ is the state manifested by the specific syndrome that consists of all the nonspecifically induced changes within a biological system; a disruption in body homeostasis and all attempts by the body to regain homeostasis.
Answer- Stress

19. _____ is a state of overstress or failure to adapt to an exercise training load.
Answer- Overtraining

Chapter 2

RESPIRATION
Outline

I. Introduction

II. Structure of the Pulmonary System

    A. The Conductive Zone

    B. The Respiratory Zone

III. Mechanics of Breathing

IV. Respiratory Circulation

V. Minute Ventilation

VI. Measurement of Lung Volumes

    A. Static Lung Volumes

    B. Dynamic Lung Volumes

    C. Spirometry

    D. Gas Dilution

    E. Standardization

VII. Partial Pressure of a Gas: Dalton's Law

VIII. Regulation of Pulmonary Ventilation

    A. The Respiratory Centers

    B. Anatomical Sensors and Factors Affecting Control of Pulmonary Ventilation

        1. Higher Brain Centers

            a. Hypothalamus

            b. Cerebral Cortex

      2. Systemic Receptors

          a. Irritant Receptors

          b. Stretch Receptors

      3. Mechanoreceptors

      4. Chemoreceptors

          a. Influence of PO_2

          b. Influence of PCO_2

          c. Influence of pH

          d. Influence of $[K^+]$

IX. Gas Exchange and Transport

    A. Gas Exchange: Henry's Law

    B. External Respiration

    C. Internal Respiration

    D. Oxygen Transport

      1. Red Blood Cells and Hemoglobin

      2. The Binding of Oxygen with Hb: The Oxygen Dissociation Curve

      3. Arteriovenous Oxygen Difference

    E. Carbon Dioxide Transport

    F. The Respiratory System and Acid-Base Balance

Chapter 2

RESPIRATION
Suggested Laboratory Activities

1. Measure static and dynamic lung volumes and have students graph and explain their results.

2. Compare and contrast the effects of hyperventilation, re-breathing of CO_2 from a bag, and exercise on breath-holding time. Relate the results to the regulatory control of respiration.

Chapter 2

Respiration
Review Questions

---

1. Define *pulmonary ventilation, external respiration,* and *internal respiration.* Define the following variables and classify each as involved in pulmonary ventilation, external respiration, or internal respiration. Some may be classified in more than one way.

       (A-a)PO$_2$diff
       a-vO$_2$ diff
       V$_D$
       f
       V$_E$ and V$_I$
       V$_T$
       PaO$_2$
       P$_A$O$_2$
       PaCO$_2$
       PvCO$_2$
       PvO$_2$
       SaO$_2$%
       SbO$_2$%
       SvO$_2$%

Figure 2.1; Pg. 21
Pulmonary ventilation is the volume of air flowing into the lungs from the external environment through either the nose or the mouth.

External respiration is the exchange of oxygen and carbon dioxide between the lungs and the blood.

Internal respiration is the exchange of oxygen and carbon dioxide at the cellular level.

Variable	Definition	Level of Involvement
(A-a)PO$_2$diff	the difference between the partial pressure of oxygen in the alveoli and the arteries	external respiration
a-vO$_2$ diff Pg. 41	arteriovenous oxygen difference: the difference between the amount of oxygen returned in venous blood and the amount originally carried in arterial blood	internal respiration
V$_D$ Pg. 22 & 26	dead space: located in the conductive zone where no exchange of gases takes place	pulmonary ventilation
f Pg. 26	frequency: the number of breaths per minute	pulmonary ventilation
V$_E$ and V$_I$ Pg. 26	minute ventilation: the amount of air inspired or expired each minute	pulmonary ventilation
V$_T$ Pg. 26	tidal volume: the amount of air inhaled or exhaled per breath	Pulmonary ventilation
P$_a$O$_2$ Pg. 31	partial pressure of oxygen in the arteries	external respiration
P$_A$O$_2$ Pg. 31	partial pressure of oxygen in the alveoli	external respiration
P$_a$CO$_2$ Pg. 31	partial pressure of carbon dioxide in the capillary	external respiration
P$_v$CO$_2$ Pg. 31	partial pressure of carbon dioxide in the venous system	internal respiration
P$_v$O$_2$ Pg. 31	partial pressure of carbon dioxide in the venous system	internal respiration
S$_a$O$_2$% Pg. 40	% saturation of oxygen in the arteries	external respiration
S$_b$O$_2$% Pg. 40	% saturation of oxygen in the blood	external respiration or internal respiration
S$_v$O$_2$% Pg. 40	% saturation of oxygen in the veins	internal respiration

2. Diagram the conductive and respiratory zones of the respiratory system. Compare the function of the two zones.

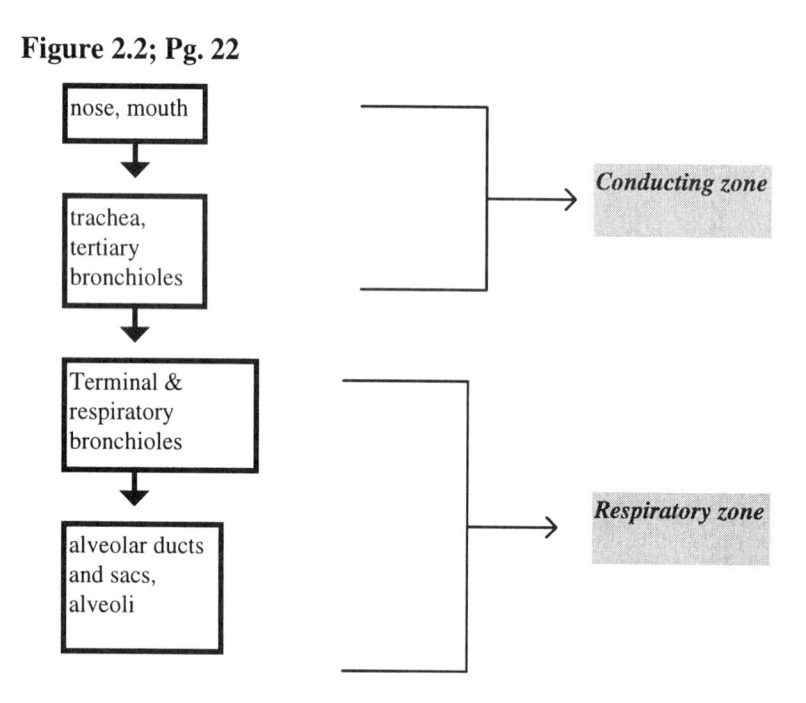

Figure 2.2; Pg. 22

```
nose, mouth
    ↓
trachea,
tertiary         ──────→ Conducting zone
bronchioles
    ↓
Terminal &
respiratory
bronchioles
    ↓                    ──────→ Respiratory zone
alveolar ducts
and sacs,
alveoli
```

3. Why does air flow into and out of the lungs?

Figure 2.3; Pgs. 23-25

Air will flow into and out of the lungs because the pressure gradients are greater than the resistance to flow. The creation of pressure gradients follows Boyle's Law as muscle activity produces changes in lung/chest volume. The following is an example: air moving out of the lungs into the atmosphere. During normal resting conditions, expiration occurs because the diaphragm and other inspirator muscles relax. When the muscles are relaxed, both the lungs and the muscles recoil to their original positions. This elastic recoil decreases lung volume, creating a pressure inside the chest cavity that is higher than the atmospheric pressure. As the chest cavity decreases in volume, the intrathoracic pressure increases slightly above that of the atmosphere. The result is that air moves out of the lungs and into the atmosphere. For air to move into the lungs (inspiration) the intercostals and the diaphragm contract, moving the ribs up and out and the diaphragm down. This action enlarges the chest cavity, and results in an increased chest volume. As a result of this increased chest volume, the chest cavity pressure is lower than atmospheric pressure and air will flow into the lungs.

Inspiration: volume increases- pressure decreases-air flows in.
Expiration: volume decreases- pressure increases- air flows out.

4. What is the functional difference between pulmonary circulation and bronchial circulation? How does bronchial circulation affect the PaO_2?

Pgs. 28-26
Pulmonary circulation serves the external respiratory function and parallels the divisions of the structures in the conductive zone.
There is a dense alveolar capillary network that covers most alveoli. This is called perfusion of the lung, which describes the capillary blood flow through this dense network.
Bronchial circulation supplies the internal respiration needs of the lung tissue and consists of relatively small systemic arteries that originate from the aorta, travel through the lungs, and return as veins that empty into the pulmonary venous system. Blood in the bronchial veins is deoxygenated and mixes with the fully oxygenated pulmonary venous blood. Because not all of the pulmonary venous blood is oxygenated, this lowers the partial pressure of oxygen in the capillaries (PaO_2).

5. Identify the three capacities and four volumes into which total lung capacity can be divided. Which of them is most responsive during exercise? Which must be accounted for when one determines body composition by hydrostatic (underwater) weighing?

Figure 2.4; Pgs. 27-28

Lung Capacity/Volume	Most responsive in exercise	Quantified for hydrostatic weighing
Tidal volume (V_T)	increases during exercise	
Inspiratory reserve volume (IRV)	decreases as V_T encroaches into it	
Expiratory reserve volume (ERV)	decreases as V_T encroaches into it	
Residual volume (RV)		Must be measured
Vital capacity (VC)		
Functional residual capacity (FRC)		
Total Lung capacity (TLC)		

6. Explain the condition represented by the volumes designations ATPS, BTPS, and STPD. Where is each condition most appropriately used? Which volume is typically the largest? Which is the smallest? Name and explain the gas laws that cause these differences?

Condition	Definition	Volume	Gas Law	Use
ATPS	*a*mbient temperature and *p*ressure, *s*aturated			Actual collection of data
BTPS	*b*ody *t*emperature, ambient *p*ressure, and fully *s*aturated with water vapor	> ATPS	**Charles's Law** (an increase in temperature will cause an increase in volume) & **Boyle's Law** (a decrease in pressure will cause an increase in volume)	lung volumes & capacity, occasionally minute ventilation ambient and body pressure are equal (both ambient) so pressure decreases because of effect of temperature on H$_2$O vapor pressure
STPD	*s*tandard *t*emperature and *p*ressure, *d*ry	< ATPS	**Charles's Law & Boyle's Law**	

7. Discuss the primary control of respiration and the factors that affect such control.

Figure 2.7; Pgs. 31-37;
There are two respiratory centers in the medulla oblongata of the brain stem (see Figure 1.8). There are also two neural centers in the pons area of the brain stem (see Figure 1.8).
The factors that affect these control centers include:
- higher brain center- hypothalamus and cerebral cortex
- system receptors
- proprioceptive receptors
- chemoreceptors

8. Describe how oxygen and carbon dioxide are transported in the circulatory system. Note in particular the importance of each transport form and any interaction between the movements of the individual gases?

Pgs. 39-43
Oxygen is carried in two ways in the blood. A small portion of the oxygen that is transported in the blood is dissolved in the plasma (liquid portion of the blood). It is this dissolved component that is responsible for the partial pressure of oxygen in the blood. The second way oxygen is transported in the blood is by being bound to hemoglobin. Approximately 97-99% of oxygen is transported in this form.

Carbon dioxide is carried three ways in the blood. A small portion of the carbon dioxide that is transported in the blood is dissolved in the blood plasma (5-10%). It is this dissolved component that is responsible for the partial pressure of carbon dioxide in the blood. The remaining 90-95% of the carbon dioxide enters the red blood cell (RBC) and 20% of this component combines chemically with the globin portion of the Hb molecule to produce the second form of carbon dioxide transport called carbamino hemoglobin. The third way that carbon dioxide is transported in the blood is as bicarbonate ions (HCO_3). Approximately 70-75% of the carbon dioxide in the RBC is transported this way.

9. Explain how the transport and removal of carbon dioxide relate to acid-base balance. Why is the maintenance of acid-base balance important?

Pg. 43
The ability of hemoglobin to bind the hydrogen ions produced during the transport of carbon dioxide and the ability of pulmonary ventilation to both respond to and eliminate carbon dioxide are important to help regulate the acid-base balance. It is important to regulate pH since all biochemical reactions in the human body require the pH to be maintained within very narrow limits for proper functioning.

10. Graph a normal resting oxygen dissociation curve. What percentage of the available oxygen is normally dissociated at rest?

   Figure 2.13; Pg. 41
   Approximately Twenty-five percent (25%) of the oxygen is released from the hemoglobin to the tissues and used during rest.

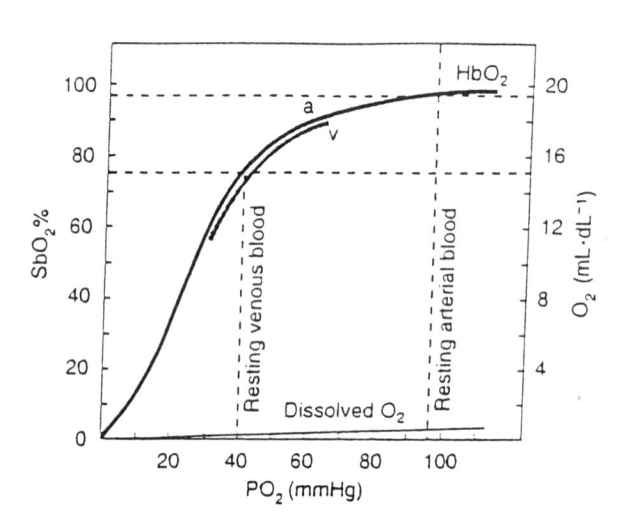

Oxygen Dissociation Curve

Chapter 2

RESPIRATION
Exam Questions

A. Multiple Choice

1. The conduction zone:
    a. warms, humidifies and filters inspired air.
    b. makes up the anatomical dead space of the respiratory system.
    c. is vulnerable to freezing if the ambient temperature is below 0^0 C.
    d. a, b, and c are correct.
    e. a and b are correct.

Answer- e

2. The respiratory zone:
    a. includes the alveoli which are the actual site of gas exchange between the pulmonary and cardiovascular systems.
    b. includes some alveoli which do not have a capillary supply and this makes up a physiological dead space.
    c. is very light weight and has a surface area as large as a badminton or tennis court over which diffusion can occur.
    d. a, b and c are correct.

Answer- d

3. Given the following information, calculate the alveolar ventilation for this individual.

    Weight - 125 lbs $P_B = 743$ mmHg
    $f = 14$ br· min^{-1} $T = 22^0$ C
    $V_T = 325$ ml· br^{-1} $P_AO_2 = 100$ mmHg

    a. 4.55 L min^{-1}
    b. 1.75 L min^{-1}
    c. 4.06 L min^{-1}
    d. 2.8 L min^{-1}

Answer- d

4. Given the following information calculate the P_{AO_2} at Pike's Peak (14,000 ft).
   P_B = 440 mmHg F_{CO_2} = .055
   F_{O_2} = .145   Water vapor pressure = 47 mmHg
   a. 103 mmHg
   b. 57 mmHg
   c. 40 mmHg
   d. 64 mmHg

Answer- b

5. Ventilation or breathing:
   a. requires that the pressure gradient must be lower than the resistance to flow.
   b. depends upon Charles's law.
   c. necessitates muscle contraction for both inspiration and expiration, even at rest.
   d. normally maintains a negative intrapleural pressure to protect the lung from collapsing.

Answer- d

6. Pulmonary circulation:
   a. furnishes blood to the lungs themselves.
   b. carries only oxygenated blood.
   c. is affected by gravity such that whatever portion of the lungs is lowest is perfused or supplied with blood best.
   d. a, b and c are correct.
   e. a and c are correct.

Answer- c

7. The static lung volume which is most responsive during exercise is:
   a. inspiratory reserve volume.
   b. tidal volume.
   c. expiratory reserve volume.
   d. residual volume.

Answer- b

8. Residual volume:
   a. represents the amount of air left in the lungs following a maximal exhalation.
   b. allows for a continuous gas exchange between breaths.
   c. must be mathematically accounted for when body composition is determined by hydrostatic (underwater) weighing.
   d. a, b, and c are correct.

Answer- d

9. When converting air volumes from the ambient conditions (ATPS) under which they were collected to standard conditions (STPD), the following law(s) should be used:

   a. Boyle's law, which states that the volume of gas is inversely related to the pressure exerted on it, if the temperature remains constant.
   b. Charles's law, which states that the volume of a gas is directly related to the temperature of the gas, if the pressure remains constant.
   c. The volume of a gas increases the higher the content of water vapor.
   d. a, b and c are correct

Answer- d

10. The inspiratory center:
    a. is cyclically active, constantly stimulated by the apneustic center, situationally inhibited by the pneumotaxic center, and stimulates the expiratory center when forceful breathing is needed.
    b. is cyclically active, situationally inhibited by the apneustic center, constantly stimulated by the pneumotaxic center and stimulates the expiratory center when forceful breathing is needed.
    c. is tonically active, constantly stimulated by both the apneustic and pneumotaxic centers to achieve a fine tuning and stimulates the expiratory center during both easy and forceful breathing.
    d. is cyclically active, situationally inhibited by both the apneustic and pneumotaxic centers to achieve fine tuning and operates totally independently of the expiratory center.

Answer- a

11. Which of the following statements is <u>not</u> true regarding factors affecting brain stem control of pulmonary ventilation?
    a. proprioceptors located in joints and muscles sensitive to bodily movement stimulate ventilation.
    b. hypothalamic sympathetic nerve system centers can either stimulate or inhibit ventilation.
    c. PO_2 is a much stronger regulator of ventilation than is PCO_2 because it affects both central and peripheral chemoreceptors.
    d. lung stretch receptors, operating as the Hering-Breuer reflex, inhibit ventilation to prevent over inflation.

Answer- c

12. Which of the following is not true regarding gas diffusion such as in external or internal respiration?
    a. Diffusion can only occur if there is a pressure gradient and the flow is from low pressure to high pressure.
    b. The rate of diffusion depends on the size of the pressure gradient, the surface area available for diffusion, the thickness of the barrier, and the solubility of the gas in the liquid.
    c. When a mixture of gases is in contact with a liquid, each gas dissolves in the liquid proportional to its partial pressure and solubility.
    d. Diffusion continues until equilibrium is achieved and the gas partial pressures are equal unless an outside factor intervenes.

Answer- a

13. Normal partial pressures of the gases involved in external respiration are:
    a. P_AO_2 = 138 mmHg; P_aO_2 = 40 mmHg; P_ACO_2 = 40 mmHg; PCO_2 = 46 mmHg
    b. P_AO_2 = 98-104 mmHg; P_aO_2 = 40 mmHg; P_ACO_2 = 40 mmHg; P_aO_2 = 46 mmHg
    c. P_AO_2 = 713 mmHg; P_aO_2 = 95 mmHg; P_ACO_2 = 713 mmHg; P_aCO_2 = 55 mmHg
    d. P_AO_2 = 98-104 mmHg; P_aO_2 = 95-96 mmHg; P_AO_2 = 40 mmHg; P_aO_2 = 40 mmHg

Answer- d

14. Given the following information calculate the a-v O_2 difference.
    dissolved a O_2 = .29 ml· dL^{-1} $S_VO_2\%$ = 45
    dissolved v O_2 = .08 ml· dL^{-1} Hb = 13 gm· dL^{-1}
    a. 9.14
    b. 9.51
    c. 4.36
    d. 10.72

Answer- b

15. Carbon dioxide is transported by the cardiovascular system.
    a. dissolved in blood plasma. The dissolved CO_2 is responsible for the P_{CO_2}.
    b. in combination with carbamino compounds, particularly the globin portion of hemoglobin.
    c. as bicarbonate ions according to the reaction $CO_2 + H_2O \rightarrow H_2CO_3 \rightarrow H^+ + HCO_3^-$; $H^+ + Hb \rightarrow HHb$.
    d. a, b and c are correct.

Answer- d

B. Fill in the Blank

1. _____ _____ is the process by which air is moved into the lungs.
   Answer- Pulmonary Ventilation

2. _____ _____ is the exchange of gases between the lungs and the blood.
   Answer- External Respiration

3. _____ _____ is the exchange of gases at the cellular level.
   Answer- Internal Respiration

4. _____ _____ is the utilization of oxygen by the cells to produce energy.
   Answer- Cellular Respiration

5. Pulmonary circulation, especially capillary blood flow is called _____ _____.
   Answer- Perfusion of the Lung

6. The amount of air inspired or expired each minute; the pulmonary ventilation rate per minute; calculated as tidal volume times frequency of breathing is called _____ _____.
   Answer- Minute Ventilation (Minute Volume) (V_I or V_E)

7. The volume of air available for gas exchange; calculated as tidal volume minus dead space volume times frequency is called _____ _____.
   Answer- Tidal Volume (V_A),

8. _____ _____ is the greatest amount of air that the lungs can contain.
   Answer- Total Lung Capacity (TLC)

9. _____ _____ is the amount of air left in the lungs following a maximal exhalation.
   Answer- Residual Volume (RV)

10. The greatest amount of air that can be exhaled following a maximal inhalation is called _____ _____.
    Answer- Vital Capacity (VC)

11. The pressure exerted by an individual gas in a mixture; determined by multiplying the fraction of the gas by the total barometric pressure is called _____ _____.
    Answer- Partial Pressure of a Gas (P_G)

12. _____ _____ is inspiration and expiration.
    Answer- Respiratory Cycle

13. _____ is normal respiration rate and rhythm.
    Answer- Eupnea

14. The tendency of gaseous, liquid, or solid molecules to move from areas of high concentration to areas of low concentration by constant random action is called _____.
    Answer- Diffusion

15. The protein portion of the red blood cell that binds with oxygen, consisting of four iron-containing pigments called hemes and a protein called globin is collectively called _____.
    Answer- Hemoglobin (Hb)

16. The ratio of the amount of oxygen combined with hemoglobin to the total oxygen capacity for combining with hemoglobin, expressed as a percentage; indicated generally as $SbO_2\%$ or specifically as $SaO_2\%$ for arterial blood or as $SvO_2\%$ for venous blood is called _____ _____.
    Answer- Percent Saturation of Hemoglobin ($SbO_2\%$)

17. The difference between the amount of oxygen returned in venous blood and the amount originally carried in arterial blood is called _____ _____.
    Answer- Arteriovenous Oxygen Difference (a-vO_2 diff)

18. The separation or release of oxygen from the red blood cells to the tissues is called _____ _____.
    Answer- Oxygen Dissociation

Chapter 3

RESPIRATORY EXERCISE RESPONSE, TRAINING ADAPTATIONS, AND SPECIAL CONSIDERATIONS
Outline

I. Response of the Respiratory System to Exercise
    A. Short-Term, Submaximal, Light-to Moderate-Intensity Dynamic Aerobic Exercise
        1. Pulmonary Ventilation
        2. External Respiration
        3. Internal Respiration
    B. Prolonged, Constant, Relatively Heavy, Submaximal Dynamic Aerobic Exercise
        1. Pulmonary Ventilation
        2. External Respiration
        3. Internal Respiration
    C. Incremental Dynamic Aerobic Exercise to Maximum
        1. Pulmonary Ventilation
        2. External Respiration
        3. Internal Respiration
    D. Static Exercise
    E. Entrainment of Respiration During Exercise

II. The Influence of Age and Sex on Respiration at Rest and During Exercise
    A. Children and Adolescents
        1. Lung Volumes and Capacities
        2. Pulmonary Ventilation
            a. Rest

    b. Submaximal Exercises

    c. maximal Exercise

   3. External and Internal Respiration

  B. The Elderly

   1. Lung Volumes and Capacities

   2. Pulmonary Ventilation

    a. Rest

    b. Submaximal Exercise

    c. Maximal Exercise

   3. External Respiration

    a. Rest

    b. Exercise

   4. Internal Respiration

  C. Male-Female Respiratory Differences

   1. Lung Volumes and Capacities

   2. Pulmonary Ventilation

   3. External and Internal Respiration

III. Respiratory Training Adaptations

  A. Lung Volumes and Capacities

  B. Pulmonary Ventilation

  C. External and Internal Respiration

  D. Why Are There So Few Respiratory Adaptations to Exercise Training?

IV. Special Considerations

  A. The Impact of Altitude on Exercise and Training

  B. Hypoxic Swim Training

  C. Exercise Training and Pollution

Chapter 3

RESPIRATORY EXERCISE RESPONSE, TRAINING ADAPTATIONS, AND SPECIAL CONSIDERATIONS
Suggested Laboratory Activities

1. Measure minute ventilation while performing the following exercises and during 5 minutes of recovery:
   - walk on the treadmill at 3.5 mi·hr^{-1} at 0% grade for 10 minutes
   - run on treadmill at 6 mi·hr^{-1} at 3% grade for 45 minutes
   - an incremental test to maximum on the treadmill
   - a static hand grip with maximal effort for 2 minutes

   Graph the results. Identify VT1 and VT2 on the appropriate graph.

2. Have each student determine whether (s)he entrains or not during a variety of rhythmical exercises.

Chapter 3

RESPIRATORY EXERCISE RESPONSE, TRAINING ADAPTATIONS, AND SPECIAL CONSIDERATIONS
Review questions

1. List and explain the four factors that increase oxygen dissociated during exercise. What venous percent saturation of oxygen (SvO2%) remains even under maximal exercise conditions?

   Figures 3.3, 3.11; pgs. 51-53, 61
   The four factors which increase oxygen dissociation during exercise are:

   1) *An increased in PO_2 gradient.* During resting conditions, the oxygen in the muscle remains at PO_2 of 40 mmHg. During exercise, the muscles utilize oxygen and PO_2 decreases, but PO_2 of arterial blood remains unchanged. Consequently, there is an increase in the pressure gradient.

   2) *An increased PCO_2.* When oxygen is used to provide energy, carbon dioxide is a byproduct. Increases in carbon dioxide will cause an increase in the PCO_2, and therefore, shifts the dissociation curve to the right. This means that more oxygen can dissociate into the muscle tissue at any given PO_2.

   3) *A decreased pH or an increased hydrogen ion concentration.* When H^+ ion increases, there is a decrease in the pH, since by definition, pH is the negative log of hydrogen concentration. This may occur in two ways: (a) CO_2 binds with water to form carbonic acid which then breaks down to hydrogen ions and bicarbonate. (b) Lactic acid also breaks down into lactate and hydrogen ions. This moves the dissociation curve to the right.

   4) *An increased temperature.* Heat, which is a byproduct of muscle energy production, is transferred from muscle tissue to the blood. This increase in temperature shifts the curve to the right. Some oxygen is always returned in the venous blood, therefore the saturation of SvO_2%, under maximal conditions, is approximately 15-35% with a partial pressure of 15-20 mmHg.

2. Compare and contrast the pulmonary ventilation, external respiration, and internal respiration responses to short-term, light to moderate submaximal exercise; long duration, heavy submaximal exercise; incremental exercise to maximum; and static exercise. Where known, explain the mechanisms for each response.

Figures 3.1, 3.2, 3.5, 3.6, 3.7, 3.8, 3.9, 3.10, 3.11; table 3.2; pgs. 49-50; Figure 2.8, pgs. 31-37

\multicolumn{4}{c	}{**Pulmonary Ventilation**}
Variables	**Comparison**	**Contrast**	**Mechanism**
V_E	Immediate triphasic response; shows a proportional increase with workload at any submaximal level, plateaus	Exhibits drift in long submaximal exercise; proportional rise is lost at ~50-75% max and again at ~85-95% max in incremental exercise; static exercise has no immediate triphasic response	An increase occurs because of changes in V_T, f, and V_D; breakpoint mechanism is unknown
V_D	decreases for all exercise levels described		Bronchodilatation
V_T	Increases rapidly and proportionally at submaximal levels below ~ 65% max, plateaus	Plateaus at ~ 60% max and then declines as maximal work is approached in incremental exercise.	Decrease in pH; an increase in $[K^+]$; chemical stimulant (chemoreceptors); sympathetic nervous stimulation; cerebral cortex (motor cortex); proprioceptice stimulation (mechanoreceptor); Figure 2.8; pgs. 31-37
f	Increases slowly and plateaus during submaximal exercise	Exhibits drift in long submaximal exercise; an exponential rise above 60% max in incremental exercise.	Same as above
V_D/V_T	Decreases initially and levels off below or at 60% max		V_T increases exceeds the decrease in V_D

External Respiration			
Variables	**Comparison**	**Contrast**	**Mechanism**
V_A	Shows proportional increase with workload at any submaximal level, plateaus	Exhibits a drift in long submaximal exercise; proportional rise is last at slightly lower %max than V_E	Parallels change in V_E
P_AO_2	Shows no change at submaximal levels below 75% max	Rises exponentially above ~75%max during incremental exercise to max.	Maintained by the increase in V_A
P_aO_2	No meaningful physiological change		Maintenance of P_AO_2 preserves driving force for oxygen transfer.
A-a (PO_2 diff)	No meaningful physiological change	Shows exponential rise above 75%max during incremental exercise to max but has no real effect	Reflects variations in P_AO_2 and ventilatory drift of V_A
$SaO_2\%$	No meaningful physiological change		Reflects maintenance of A-a(PO_2diff)

Internal Respiration			
Variables	**Comparison**	**Contrast**	**Mechanism**
P_aCO_2	Is level and then decreases slightly		CO_2 is blown off with increased hyperpnea of exercise
P_VCO_2	Rises proportionally to workload		The increase in energy production results in the increase of CO_2 as a by-product
P_VO_2	Decreases proportionally to workload		The increase in energy production results in the increased oxygen use
S_VO_2	Decreases proportionally to workload		The increase in energy production results in the increased oxygen use
a-vO_2diff	Shows a proportional increase with submaximal workloads below ~40-60% max then plateaus	Exhibits drift in long submaximal exercise; plateaus at 40-60% max during incremental exercise to maximum in all but highly trained individuals	The increase in energy production results in the increased oxygen use

3. Should fitness participants and athletes be encouraged to practice entrainment as opposed to spontaneous breathing? Why or why not?

> **Pgs. 61, 63**
> A person who engages in a physical fitness program should breathe whenever it is most natural. It has been noted that individuals who participate in natural entrainment have a lower energy cost during exercise. However, it was also noted that individuals who are forced into entrainment patterns do not share the results of having lower energy cost. If the individual is participating in a weight program, he/she should entrainment breathing **specifically**, exhaling during the lifting portion of the contraction. This will reduce the chances of experiencing the Valsalva maneuver, which is abnormally high blood pressure resulting from the breath being held against a closed glottis.

4. Explain exercise-induced hypoxemia (EIH) and discuss why it occurs only in highly trained elite athletes. Relate the factors responsible for EIH to the low incidence of respiratory training adaptations.

> **Figures 3.10, 3,11; pgs. 58-59, 70**
> Exercise Induced Hypoxemia (EIH) is a condition that occurs in about 40-50% of elite male athletes in which there is insufficient oxygenation of the blood. The ability to process oxygen and perform high intensity performance for these athletes are lowered, although they still exceed those of untrained individuals. Possible causes for EIH include the inequality between ventilation and perfusion, and a limitation in diffusion. Failure to achieve complete diffusion equilibrium may be related to the faster transit time of RBC through lung capillaries. In sedentary or moderately trained individuals, pulmonary capillary blood volume increases during exercise. This increases the surface area for diffusion and slows down RBC transit time. In highly trained athletes, pulmonary capillary blood volume and hence surface area reach their maximum at relatively low workloads. If the workload and total body circulation continue to increase, so does blood flow velocity. This decreases the time RBC are in the pulmonary capillaries and diffusion is limited. External respiration is a limitation factor in these cases. There is a low incidence in respiratory training adaptations because the adaptations in the cardiovascular and metabolic systems usually do not go beyond the capability of the respiratory system. Athletes with EIH illustrate an exception to this rule.

5. Prepare a flowchart of the physiological changes that occur as a result of acute exposure to altitude. How are these acute changes modified by acclimatization?

Pgs. 70-73

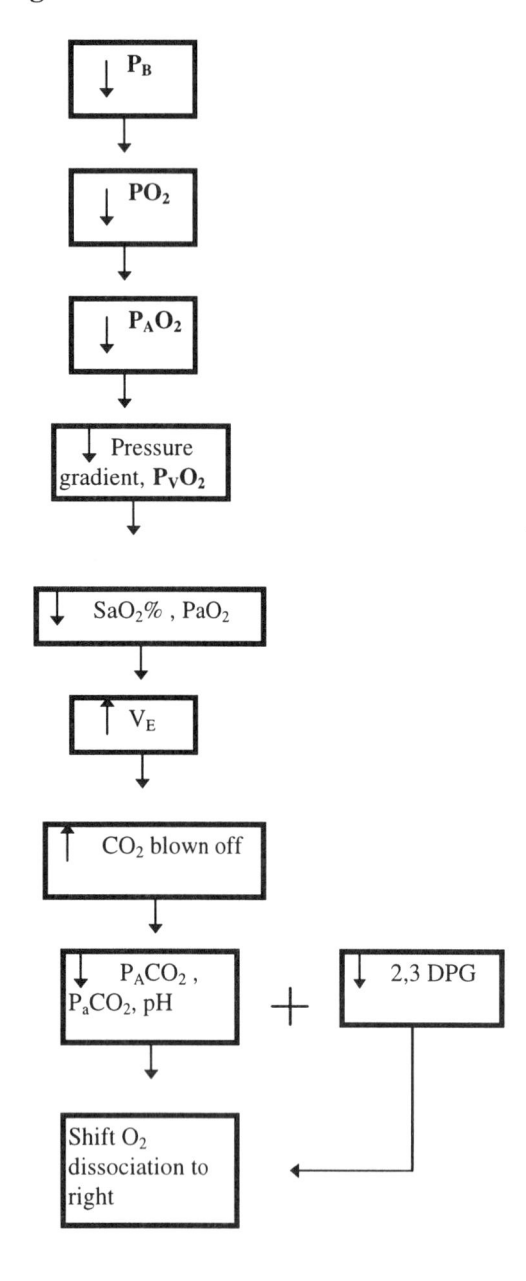

```
↓ P_B
  ↓
↓ PO_2
  ↓
↓ P_AO_2
  ↓
↓ Pressure gradient, P_VO_2
  ↓
↓ SaO_2%, PaO_2
  ↓
↑ V_E
  ↓
↑ CO_2 blown off
  ↓
↓ P_ACO_2, P_aCO_2, pH     +     ↓ 2,3 DPG
  ↓                                 ↓
Shift O_2 dissociation to right ←──┘
```

Acute
- There is an increase in Hb concentration which will increase the amount of O_2 transported
- Initially due to hemoconcentration; a result of a decrease in BV that leads to an increase in viscosity and resistance, that results in an increased HR

Acclimatization
- There is an increase in Hb concentration RBC + BV increase (reversal of acute changes)
- Hyperventilation maintained
- Increase in VT not f
- Increase in VT allows for a more effective gas exchange
- PaO2 increases

6. Defend or refute this statement: "Hypoxic training, whether achieved by training at altitude or breath holding is beneficial to the athlete."

Pgs. 72-73
There does not appear to be any advantage over and above that gained from exercise training itself. The only advantage of altitude training is if the event is at altitude. Generally, training volume (especially intensity) cannot be maintained at altitude.

Breath holding while swimming does not produce hypoxia, but hypercapnia. Thus, even if hypoxia was beneficial to training, it would not result from controlled frequency breathing in swimming.

Chapter 3

RESPIRATORY EXERCISE RESPONSE, TRAINING ADAPTATIONS, AND SPECIAL CONSIDERATIONS
Exam Questions

A. Multiple Choice

1. Hyperventilation:
   a. increases the P_aO_2
   b. decreases the P_aCO_2
   c. if combined with underwater swimming can lead to fatalities since an individual can continue patterned motor activity after loss of consciousness caused by lack of oxygen to the brain.
   d. a, b, and c are correct.
   e. b and c are correct.

Answer- e

2. Respiration (pulmonary ventilation, external respiration and/or internal respiration) is a limiting factor in maximal exercise in:
   a. children and adolescents.
   b. sedentary middle aged adults.
   c. highly trained elite male cyclists and runners.
   d. elderly moderately fit female swimmers.

Answer- c

3. The basic pattern of response to all exercise modalities is the same for males and females, except:
   a. at the same submaximal ventilation during aerobic exercise, females display a higher tidal volume and lower breathing frequency than males.
   b. at maximal aerobic exercise, males exhibit higher minute ventilation than females.
   c. males show larger a-vO_2 differences than do females during submaximal and maximal aerobic exercise.
   d. during dynamic resistance activity, females show greater a-vO_2 differences than do males.

Answer- b

4. Given the following information calculate the a-v O_2 difference.
   dissolved a O_2 = .29 ml· dL^{-1} $S_VO_2\%$ = 45
   dissolved v O_2 = .14 ml· dL^{-1} Hb = 13 gm· dL^{-1}
   a. 9.14
   b. 9.29
   c. 4.36
   d. 10.72

Answer-

5. Exercise induced hypoxemia:
   a. has been reported only in some highly trained elite male runners and cyclists.
   b. is exhibited as a sharp and meaningful increase in P_aO_2, $SaO_2\%$ and (A-a) PO_2 diff.
   c. is probably caused by a red blood cell transit time through the pulmonary circuit that is too fast to allow for adequate diffusion and the achievement of gas equilibrium.
   d. a, b and c are correct.
   e. a and c are correct.

Answer- e

6. The synchronization of limb movement and breathing frequency:
   a. results in a lower energy cost during exercise.
   b. should be recommended for beginning exercisers in jogging and stair stepping programs.
   c. should be coordinated for weight lifters such that inhalation should occur during the lowering phase of a resistance exercise and exhalation during the lifting phase of each repetition.
   d. a, b and c are correct.

Answer- c

7. Respiratory adaptations to aerobic exercise training:
   a. indicate that while land-based activities may cause changes in specific static lung volumes and capacities, especially vital capacity, water-based activities do not.
   b. are most consistent as an increase in V_E L· min^{-1} during submaximal work and an increase at maximum.
   c. include a decrease in the a-vO_2 difference at maximal exercise in young adults.
   d. are few and inconsistent, probably because the tremendous reserve capacity means the various components are not stressed and so do not need to change.

Answer- d

8. Altitude:
   a. affects the P_aO_2 because while the percentage of oxygen in air remains constant at 20.93%, the barometric pressure decreases exponentially.
   b. causes hyperventilation, a decrease in P_ACO_2 and P_aCO_2, hemoconcentration, and an increase in heart rate.
   c. causes a decrease in performance for aerobic endurance, anaerobic sprint, and muscular power athletes.
   d. a, b, and c are correct.
   e. a and b are correct.

Answer- e

9. Altitude training:
   a. can and should be carried out at the same level of intensity, duration and frequency in order to maximize its benefits.
   b. is most beneficial to those athletes who suffer from exercise induced hypoxemia (EIH).
   c. is additive, that is, the benefits achieved are over and above those which training alone would have caused for most individuals.
   d. is most beneficial if it occurs at the same altitude and immediately precedes a competition at altitude not sea level.

Answer- d

10. Hypoxic swim training:
    a. reduces the volume of air taken in by the swimmer and creates hypoxia which is beneficial to the swimmer's training.
    b. involves controlled frequency breathing which produces hypercapnia or an increase in P_aCO_2.
    c. involves controlled frequency breathing which increases buoyancy and improves body position.
    d. a, b and c are correct.
    e. b and c are correct.

Answer- e

11. Which of the following statements are correct?
    a. A 4% COHb level will have a detrimental effect on exercise time and intensity because CO binds to the same site on hemoglobin as oxygen would, thus decreasing SaO_2%.
    b. An individual who smokes 10 or fewer cigarettes per day averages 4% COHb while a two pack a day smoker averages almost 8% COHb.
    c. Nonsmokers riding in a car for 1 hour with a smoker can reach 3% COHb.
    d. a, b and c are correct.

Answer- d

12. The pattern of response to aerobic submaximal and incremental exercise to maximum is similar between children/adolescents and young/middle aged adults except:
    a. children exhibit a higher breathing frequency and lower tidal volume at any given submaximal load than young or middle aged adults.
    b. children/adolescents do not exhibit the ventilatory breakpoints during incremental exercise to maximum.
    c. children/adolescents cannot extract as much oxygen during maximal exercise as young/middle aged adults do.
    d. a, b, and c are correct.

Answer- a

13. The pattern of response to aerobic submaximal and incremental exercise to maximum is similar between the elderly and young/middle aged adults except:
    a. the elderly exhibit a higher minute ventilation at any given submaximal workload than young/middle aged adults.
    b. the ventilatory breakpoints occur at lower absolute and relative workloads in the elderly compared with young/middle aged adults.
    c. maximal minute ventilation is lower in the elderly than in young/middle aged adults.
    d. a, b, and c are correct.

Answer- d

14. In order to minimize the impact of pollutants upon exercise training or competition, individuals:
    a. should not try to adapt to breathing pollutants because this can suppress normal defense mechanisms.
    b. should exercise at least 50 feet from motor vehicles.
    c. should schedule workouts mid-afternoon to early evenings to avoid the peak hours of pollution.
    d. a, b, and c are correct.
    e. a and b are correct.

Answer- e

15. The breaks in linearity of $\dot{V}_E$ with incremental exercise to max are most accurately labeled:
    a. lactate thresholds
    b. aerobic thresholds
    c. pulmonary thresholds
    d. ventilatory thresholds

Answer- d

16. Which of the following statements is <u>not</u> accurate regarding respiration in normal healthy, sedentary or moderately fit individuals?
    a. Pulmonary ventilation increases in response to exercise to enhance alveolar ventilation.
    b. External respiration adjusts in such a way as to maintain the relationship between ventilation and perfusion in response to exercise.
    c. Internal respiration responds to exercise with increased extraction of oxygen by the muscles.
    d. Respiration can be considered a limitation to maximal work.

Answer- d

B. Fill in the Blank

1. Increased pulmonary ventilation that matches an increased metabolic demand, as in an exercise situation, is referred to as _____.
   Answer- Hyperpnea

2. _____ _____ are points where the rectilinear rise in minute ventilation breaks from linearity during an incremental exercise to maximum.
   Answer- Ventilatory Thresholds

3. A condition found in elite male endurance athletes in which the amount of oxygen carried in arterial blood is severely reduced is _____ _____ _____.
   Answer- Exercise-Induced Hypoxemia

4. The synchronization of limb movement and breathing frequency that accompanies rhythmical exercise is _____.
   Answer- Entrainment

5. Breath-holding that involves closing of the glottis and contraction of the diaphragm and abdominal musculature is called the _____ _____.
   Answer- Valsalva Maneuver

6. Increased pulmonary ventilation, especially ventilation that exceeds metabolic requirements; carbon dioxide is blown off, leading to a decrease in its partial pressure in arterial blood. This condition is called _____.
   Answer- Hyperventilation

THE CARDIOVASCULAR SYSTEM
Outline

I. Introduction

II. Overview of the Cardiovascular System

    A. The Heart

        1. Macroanatomy of the Heart

        2. Microanatomy of the Heart

        3. The Heart as Excitable Tissue

        4. Electrocardiogram

        5. Cardiac Cycle

        6. Stroke Volume

        7. Cardiac Output

        8. Coronary Circulation

        9. Myocardial Oxygen Consumption

    B. The Vascular System

        1. Arteries

        2. Arterioles

        3. Capillaries

        4. Venules

        5. Veins

    C. Blood

    D. Hormonal Control of Blood Volume

III. Cardiovascular Dynamics

    A. Cardiac Output (Q)

    B. Principles of Blood Flow

IV. Regulation of the Cardiovascular System

    A. Neural Control

    B. Anatomical Sensors and Factors Affecting Control of the Cardiovascular System

        1. Higher Brain Centers

        2. Systemic Receptors

            a. Baroreceptors

            b. Stretch Receptors

        3. Chemoreceptors

        4. Muscle Joint Receptors

    C. Neuro-hormonal Control

V. Assessment of Cardiovascular Variables

    A. Cardiac Output

    B. Stroke Volume

    C. Heart Rate

    D. Maximal Oxygen Consumption

        1. Factors Limiting VO_2max

        2. Heritability of VO_2max

        3. Field Tests of Cardiorespiratory Capacity (VO_2max)

    E. Blood Pressure

Chapter 4

THE CARDIOVASCULAR SYSTEM
Suggested Laboratory Activities

1. Practice measuring:
    - heart rate by auscultation over the heart and by palpation at the radial and carotid sites
    - blood pressure by auscultation

   Calculate mean arterial blood pressure and rate pressure product from the results.

2. Take an ECG and compute heart rate

3. Complete a field test of cardiorespiratory capacity

Chapter 4

THE CARDIOVASCULAR SYSTEM
Review Questions

1. Diagram the conducting system of the heart, and describe how activation of the SA node leads to contraction of the heart.

Figure 4.3; pgs. 82-83

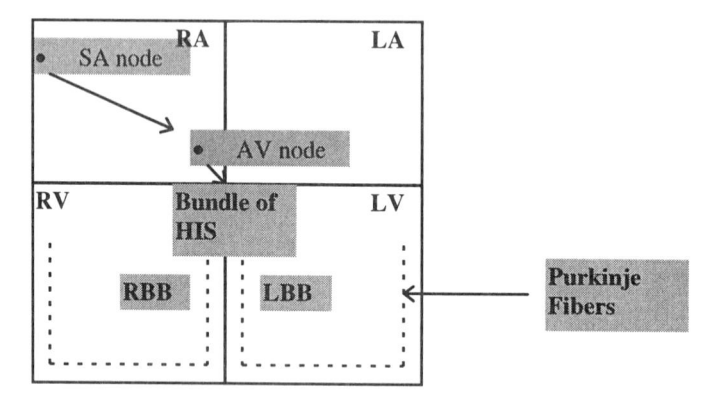

	RA	LA	
	• SA node		
		• AV node	
RV		Bundle of HIS	LV
	RBB	LBB	← Purkinje Fibers

Once depolarization of the pacemaker cell (SA node) occurs, this electrical activity spreads to the AV node, then to the bundle of HIS, then to the left and right bundle branches, then onto the Purkinje Fibers. This excites the myocardial cells. Excitation of myocardial cells is spread cell to cell causing all the cells of the ventricles to contract.

2. Describe the electrical events in the heart in relationship to pressure in the left ventricle, the volume of blood in the left ventricle, and the position of the heart valves.

Figure 4.5; pgs. 84-87

The P wave reflects atrial depolarization. At this time there is little pressure in the ventricles because they are relaxed (ventricular diastole). Ventricular blood volume is increasing because the AV valves are open, allowing blood that is returned to the heart to flow from the atria into the ventricles (VEP). Atrial contraction will also push additional blood into the ventricles at the end of this diastole phase. The QRS wave reflects ventricular contraction (systole).

Ventricular pressure increases rapidly and dramatically as the ventricles contract. Initially, ventricular volume remains unchanged (ICP) because the semilunar valves are closed. When ventricular pressure exceeds aortic pressure, the semilunar valves are pushed open and ventricular volume falls sharply as blood is ejected from the ventricles (VEP). Once pressure in the aorta exceeds left ventricular pressure, the semilunar valves close and T wave results from ventricular repolarization. Thus, the ventricles are at rest (diastole) and pressure is low. As the AV valves open, the ventricles begin to fill with blood, thereby increasing blood volume in the ventricles markedly and ventricular pressure slightly.

3. Identify the different vessels of the peripheral circulation, and describe the velocity and pressure in each. What accounts for the differences?

Figure 4.12; pgs. 90-94, 97-98
The vessels of the peripheral circulation include: arteries, arterioles, capillaries, venules and veins. The arteries are thick walled conduits that carry blood from the heart to the various organs, while the arterioles are smaller than the arteries and are the major site or resistance in the vascular system. The capillaries perform the ultimate function of the cardiovascular system: exchanging gases and nutrients between the blood and tissues. The venules are small vessels on the venous side of the vascular system, and the veins (capacitance vessels) serve as low-resistance conduits that return blood to the heart. The velocity of blood flow is inversely related to the total cross sectional area of the vessels. The velocity of the blood is greatest in the arteries due to the small total cross sectional area of the arteries and the force of ventricular contraction. The velocity of blood flow decreases dramatically as blood flows through the arterioles (resistance vessels), reaching its slowest velocity in the capillaries (allowing adequate time for gas exchange). Blood velocity increases in the venules and veins as total cross section area is much smaller than in the capillaries (Fig. 4.12b). Blood pressure is greatest in the aorta and decreases progressively as the blood travels through the vascular tree, reaching it's lowest level of approximately 0-4 mmHg in the great veins and the right atrium.

4. Describe the hormonal mechanisms by which the body attempts to compensate for a decrease in plasma volume.

> **Figure 4.11; pgs. 95-96**
> A reduction in blood volume is associated with an increase in blood osmolarity. This increase in osmolarity of the blood stimulates osmoreceptors in the hypothalamus which signals the posterior pituitary gland to release ADH. The ADH causes the kidneys to retain water and leads to the increase in blood volume. A decrease in blood volume also leads to a decrease in the blood pressure in the atrium and arteries. The activation of the atrial baroreceptors and arterial receptors (in the kidneys) lead to the release of ADH which causes the tubules in the kidneys to reabsorb the water to increase blood volume. Additionally, receptors in the kidneys respond to the decrease in arterial pressure by releasing renin, an enzyme necessary for the conversion of angiotensin II. Angiotension II then signals the adrenal cortex to release aldosterone, causing the kidneys to retain salt and water. Angiotensin II also has a vasoconstrictor affect on arterioles, increasing blood pressure.

5. Discuss the neurohumoral regulation of the cardiovascular system and the factors that affect such regulation.

> **Figure 4.14; pgs. 98-100**
> The sympathetic and parasympathetic outflow from the cardiovascular centers in the medullar are influenced by the following factors:
> 1) <u>Influence of the higher brain centers</u>: Input from the cerebral cortex and the hypothalamus affect cardiovascular centers in the medulla. Emotions influence cardiovascular function at rest. Motor cortex input can increase HR and cause vasodilatation during exercise. Body temperature influences cardiovascular centers resulting in increased HR and vasodilation.
> 2) <u>Systemic receptors:</u> *Baroreceptors* located in the aorta and carotid bodies are sensitive to an increase in MAP and cause a reflex decrease in MAP due to decrease in HR. *Stretch receptors* located in the right atrium. An increase in venous return stretches theses receptors causing an increase in cardiac output. This response is known as the Bainbridge reflex
> 3) <u>Chemoreceptors</u>: Are found in the aorta and carotid arteries and are sensitive to PO_2, PCO_2, and H^+. An increase in PCO_2, and H^+, or a decrease in PCO_2 causes a reflex vasoconstriction of arterioles.

4) <u>Muscle receptors</u>: *Mechanoreceptors* and *metaboreceptors* are found in the joints and muscles. These receptors sends impulses to the brain which leads to an increase rate and force of heart contraction and vasodilation in active muscle.

6. Why is maximal oxygen consumption (VO$_2$max) considered to be a cardiovascular variable?

Pgs. 103-104
The assessment of VO$_2$max provides a means for quantifying the functional capacity of the entire cardiovascular system. The role of the cardiovascular system in determining VO$_2$max can be seen in the following equation: VO$_2$max = Q max X a-vO$_2$diff max .

7. What are the possible factors limiting maximal oxygen consumption? What are the most likely factors limiting it?

Pg. 104
Maximal oxygen consumption may be limited by the ability of the a) respiratory system to take in oxygen, b) cardiovascular system to transport oxygen, or c) skeletal muscles to extract and utilize oxygen. The functional capacity of the respiratory system exceeds the demands of maximal exercise in normal, healthy individuals without EIH. The skeletal muscles posses a greater ability to use oxygen then can be supplied by the respiratory and cardiovascular system. Thus, cardiovascular factors are most likely to limit VO$_2$max. Oxygen uptake is not a limiting factor in VO$_2$max in normal, healthy (non)/athletes without EIH. The cardiovascular system is the primary system limiting oxygen consumption in individuals.

8. Explain the steps involved in attaining an accurate measurement of blood pressure.

Figure 4.18; Pgs. 106-107
Have the subject rest quietly. Properly place the cuff around the upper arm. Inflate the cuff to about 140 mmHg during rest. Slowly deflate the cuff at a rate of 2-3 mmHg per second and listen closely for the first sound (Korotkoff sound). This first sound is the systolic blood pressure. The disappearance of the sound (5th Korotkoff sound) is the diastolic blood pressure. The muffling of the sound (4th Korotkoff sound) is recorded as the DBP for children and during exercise. Release the pressure and remove the cuff.

Chapter 4

THE CARDIOVASCULAR SYSTEM
Exam Questions

A. Multiple Choice

1. Place the following in sequence for a normal cardiac cycle beginning with atrial systole.
    1. Atrial systole
    2. Isovolumetric relaxation period
    3. Ventricular ejection period
    4. Atrial and ventricular diastole and filling
    5. Isovolumetric contraction period
        a. 1, 4, 2, 5, 3
        b. 1, 5, 3, 2, 4
        c. 1, 3, 4, 5, 2
        d. 1, 2, 3, 4, 5

Answer- b

2. Place the following in sequence for normal ECG conduction:
    1. Purkinje fibers
    2. S-A Node
    3. Bundle branches
    4. anterior internodal pathway & Bachmann's bundle
    5. A-V Node
    6. Bundle of His
        a. 1, 2, 3, 4, 5, 6
        b. 2, 5, 6, 3, 1, 4
        c. 2, 4, 5, 6, 3, 1
        d. 2, 5, 4, 3, 6, 1

Answer- c

3. Which of the following is a principle governing blood flow?
   a. Blood pressure flows through the vessels of the circulatory system because resistance is greater than pressure gradient.
   b. Different volumes of blood must pass each and any point (vessel type) in the circulatory system per unit of time to adjust for differences in vessel diameters.
   c. The velocity of blood flow past any point varies inversely with the total cross-sectional area of the vascular bed at that point; where the total cross-sectional area is larger, the velocity is slower and vise versa.
   d. The less viscous the fluid, the greater the resistance to its flow.

Answer- c

4. An individual has an exercise blood pressure of 150/70/60 mmHg, a heart rate of 140 b·min^{-1}, O$_2$ consumption of 33 ml·kg^{-1}·min^{-1} and a stroke volume of 95 ml·beat^{-1}. What is his mean arterial blood pressure?
   a. 90 mmHg
   b. 96.4 mmHg
   c. 105 mmHg
   d. 110 mmHg

Answer- d

5. What is this individual's (in question #4) cardiac output?
   a. 9.5 L·min^{-1}
   b. 13.3 L·min^{-1}
   c. 14.3 L·min^{-1}
   d. 15.8 L·min^{-1}

Answer- b

6. What is the resistance to the flow of blood under these conditions in this individual (in question #4)? [no units are needed]
   a. 16.67
   b. 11.6
   c. 8.27
   d. 7.14

Answer- c

7. Place the following in the proper sequence for a normal action potential:
   1. [K+] highest inside; [Na+] highest outside; - charge inside
   2. propagation down length of nerve
   3. Na+ influx; + charge inside
   4. K+ efflux; - charge inside
      a. 1, 2, 3, 4,
      b. 3, 1, 4, 2
      c. 1, 3, 4, 2
      d. 1, 4, 2, 3

Answer- c

8. Factors which provide sensory or afferent information to the cardio accelerator, cardio inhibitory and vasomotorcenters and predominate in achieving the exercise response include:
   a. stretch receptors responding to increased venous return.
   b. baroreceptors responding to increased mean arterial blood pressure.
   c. mechanoreceptors or proprioceptors responding to muscle movement.
   d. a, b, and c are correct.
   e. a and c are correct.

Answer- e

9. Stimulation of the accelerator nerve to the heart results in:
   a. an increased force of contraction.
   b. a decreased excitability and conductivity.
   c. an increased rate of contraction.
   d. a, b, and c are correct.
   e. a and c are correct.

Answer- e

10. Which of the following is not a principle governing blood flow?
    a. Blood pressure flows through the vessels of the circulatory system because of differences in pressure.
    b. The same volume of blood must pass each and any point (vessel type) in the circulatory system per unit of time.
    c. The velocity of blood flow past any point depends upon the total cross-sectional area of the vascular bed at that point; where the total cross-sectional area is larger, the velocity must be higher and vise versa.
    d. The more viscous the fluid, the greater the resistance to its flow.

Answer- c

11. Which of the following is/are an important mechanism(s) for increasing the blood flow to active skeletal muscles during exercise?
    a. vasodilation mediated by sympathetic nerve endings and the neurotransmitter acetylcholine
    b. muscle contraction and relaxation
    c. the action of metabolites such as phosphates, potassium, and lactic acid
    d. b, and c are correct

Answer- d

12. Stroke volume (in untrained individuals):
    a. increases with an increase in end-diastolic volume (EDV) up to about 250 ml and then decreases slightly with any further increase in EDV.
    b. decreases at any given end-diastolic volume under the influence of sympathetic nerve stimulation, epinephrine or norepinephrine.
    c. increases rectilinearly with end-diastolic volume throughout the range of values.
    d. increases rectilinearly under the influence of sympathetic nerve stimulation, epinephrine or norepinephrine throughout the range of motion.

Answer- a

13. A slowed heart beat is called:
    a. murmur
    b. flutter
    c. bradycardia
    d. tachycardia

Answer- c

14. Baroreceptors are sensitive to:
    a. an increase in resistance and decrease in pH.
    b. an increase in MAP.
    c. a decrease in DBP and HR.
    d. a decrease in parasympathetic outflow.

Answer-b

15. As the ventricles contracts:
    a. pressure inside the ventricles decreases rapidly.
    b. pressure inside the ventricles stays the same.
    c. pressure inside the ventricles increases dramatically.
    d. Myocardium contraction doesn't affect pressure.

Answer- c

16. Cardiovascular drift is evidenced by a:
    a. decreased SV.
    b. decreased HR.
    c. higher maximal work value
    d. decreased SBP

Answer- a

17. Rate pressure product is calculated as:
    a. HR x DBP
    b. SV x Q
    c. HR x SBP
    d. HR x SV

Answer- c

18. The T wave reflects:
    a. atrial depolarization
    b. ventricle depolarization
    c. ventricle repolarization
    d. atrial repolarization

Answer- c

19. Which statement is true regarding cardiovascular dynamics?
    a. velocity decreases as total cross sectional area increases
    b. velocity increases as total cross sectional area increases
    c. velocity remains the same as total cross sectional area increases
    d. none of the above

Answer- a

20. Resistance can be calculated as:
    a. TPR / Q
    b. Q / SV
    c. MAP / HR
    d. MAP / Q

Answer- d

21. The atrio-ventricualr valves:
    a. lead to systemic circulation
    b. lead to pulmonary circulation
    c. separate the atria and ventricles
    d. prevent blood from flowing backward

Answer-c

22. Under resting conditions, the heart ejects about _____% of the blood that is returned:
   a. 10-20
   b. 30-40
   c. 50-60
   d. 70-80

Answer- c

23. Found in the right atria, the conduction-system cells with the fastest spontaneous rate of depolarization:
   a. Purkinje fibers
   b. bachmans bundle
   c. SA node
   d. RBCs

Answer- c

24. The exchange of gases and nutrients in the capillaries depends on:
   a. osmosis
   b. diffusion
   c. nutrients
   d. VO$_2$ max

Answer- b

25. Forcibly exhaling against a closed glottis is called the:
   a. Valsalva maneuver
   b. pressor response
   c. impossible
   d. contraction phase of inspiration

Answer- a

26. The _____ represents the electrical activity of the muscle cells:
   a. myocardium
   b. pressure (mmHg)
   c. ECG
   d. syncytium

Answer- c

27. Individual cells of the myocardium function collectively; the functionally collective unit is called:
   a. intercalated discs
   b. myosin
   c. actin
   d. syncytium

Answer- c

28. The SA node normally contracts _____ times per minute.
   a. 40-60
   b. 75-80
   c. 85-100
   d. 15-45

Answer- b

B.   Fill in the Blank

1. The junction between cardiac muscle cells that forms the mechanical and electrical connection between the two cells are the _____ _____.
   Answer- Intercalated Discs

2. _____ is the individual cells of the myocardium functioning collectively as a unit during depolarization.
   Answer- Syncytium

3. One complete sequence of contraction and relaxation of the heart is called the _____ _____.
   Answer- Cardiac Cycle

4. _____ _____ _____ _____ _____ is defined as the volume of blood in the left ventricle at the end of diastole.
   Answer- Left Ventricular End-Diastolic Volume

5. The volume of blood in the left ventricle at the end of systole is the _____ _____ _____ _____ _____ _____.
   Answer- Left Ventricular End-Systolic Volume

6. _____ _____ is the amount of blood ejected from the ventricles with each beat of the heart.
   Answer- Stroke Volume

7. _____ _____ is the number of cardiac cycles per minute, expressed as beats per min (b·min^{-1}).
   Answer- Heart Rate

8. The volume of blood returned to the heart is known as _____ of the heart.
   Answer- Preload

9. The percentage of LVEDV that is ejected from the heart is the _____ _____.
   Answer- Ejection Fraction

10. The force of contraction of the heart is termed _____.
    Answer- Contractility

11. Resistance presented to the contracting ventricle is a definition for _____.
    Answer- Afterload

12. The amount of blood pumped per unit of time is the _____ _____.
    Answer- Cardiac Output

13. The force exerted on the wall of the blood vessel by the blood as a result of contraction of the heart (systole) or relaxation of the heart (diastole) is called _____ _____.
    Answer- Blood Pressure

14. _____ _____ can change their diameter allowing them to control the flow of blood.
    Answer- Resistance Vessels

15. _____ _____ are another name for veins, owing to their distensibility, which enables them to pool large volumes of blood and become reservoirs for blood.
    Answer- Capacitance Vessels

16. _____ is defined as the ratio of blood cells to total blood volume, expressed as a percentage.
    Answer- Hematocrit

17. _____ is opposition to blood flow.
    Answer- Resistance

18. The _____ _____ is an equation used to calculate cardiac output from oxygen consumption and arteriovenous oxygen difference (a-vO_2 diff).
    Answer- Fick Equation

19. _____ _____ is a technique that calculates stroke volume form measurements of aortic cross-sectional area and time-velocity integrals in the ascending aorta.
    Answer- Doppler Echocardiography

CARDIOVASCULAR RESPONSES TO EXERCISE
Outline

I. Introduction

II. Cardiovascular Responses to Dynamic Aerobic Exercise

    A. Short Term, Submaximal, Light to Moderate Intensity Exercise

    B. Prolonged, Heavy, Submaximal Dynamic Exercise

    C. Incremental Dynamic Exercise to Maximum

    D. Upper- Body versus Lower-Body Exercise

    E. Sex Differences During Dynamic Aerobic Exercise

        1. Submaximal Exercise

        2. Incremental Exercise to Maximum

    F. Responses of Children to Dynamic Aerobic Exercise

        1. Submaximal Exercise

        2. Incremental Exercise to Maximum

    G. Responses of Elderly to Dynamic Aerobic Exercise

        1. Submaximal Exercise

        2. Incremental Exercise to Maximum

III. Cardiovascular Responses to Static Exercise
    A. Intensity of Muscle Contraction
        1. Blood Flow During Static Contractions
        2. Comparison of Dynamic Aerobic and Static Exercise
    B. Sex Differences in Responses to Static Exercise
    C. Cardiovascular Response to Static Exercise in Older Adults

IV. Cardiovascular Responses to Dynamic Resistance Exercise

Chapter 5

CARDIOVASCULAR RESPONSE TO EXERCISE
Suggested Laboratory Activities

1. Measure heart rate and blood pressure while the following exercises are performed and during 5 minutes of recovery:
    - walk on the treadmill at 3.5 mi·hr^{-1} at 0% grade for 10 minutes
    - run on the treadmill at 6 mi·hr^{-1} for 45 minutes
    - an incremental test to maximum on the treadmill
    - a static handgrip with maximal effort for 3 minutes
    - 1 set of 8 reps at 75% 1-RM of 2 arm biceps curls

Graph the results. Compute mean arterial pressure and rate pressure product and graph these results.

2. Determine maximal oxygen consumption from a variety of protocols and on a variety of modes of exercise.

Chapter 5

CARDIOVASCULAR RESPONSE TO EXERCISE
Review Questions

1. Graph and explain the pattern of response for each of the major cardiovascular variables during short term, light to moderate dynamic aerobic exercise. Explain the mechanisms responsible for each response.

Figure 5.1; Table 5.1; pgs. 112-115

Variable	Pattern of Response	Mechanism
Cardiac Output	Increases rapidly, levels off at steady state within two minutes of exercise	Due to the increase in both stroke volume and heart rate
Stroke Volume	Increases rapidly, levels off at steady state within two minutes of exercise	Due to an increase in venous return. This increase in venous return increases LVEDV (preload). This increase in preload will increase contractility of the myocardium as well as the increased sympathetic nervous system. There is also a decrease in LVESV.
Heart Rate	Increases rapidly, levels off at steady state within two minutes of exercise	Due to a withdrawal of the parasympathetic nervous system.
Systolic Blood Pressure	Increases rapidly, levels off at steady state within two minutes of exercise	Due to the increase in cardiac output.
Diastolic Blood Pressure	No change	Due to the peripheral vasodilation which facilitates blood flow to the working muscles.
Mean Arterial Pressure	Increases rapidly, levels off at steady state within two minutes of exercise	Due to the changes in SBP and DBP.
Total Peripheral Resistance	No change	Due to the vasodilation of the active muscles.
Rate Pressure Product	Increases rapidly, levels off at steady state within two minutes of exercise	The change is due to increases in both heart rate and SBP, showing a greater myocardial oxygen demand of the heart.

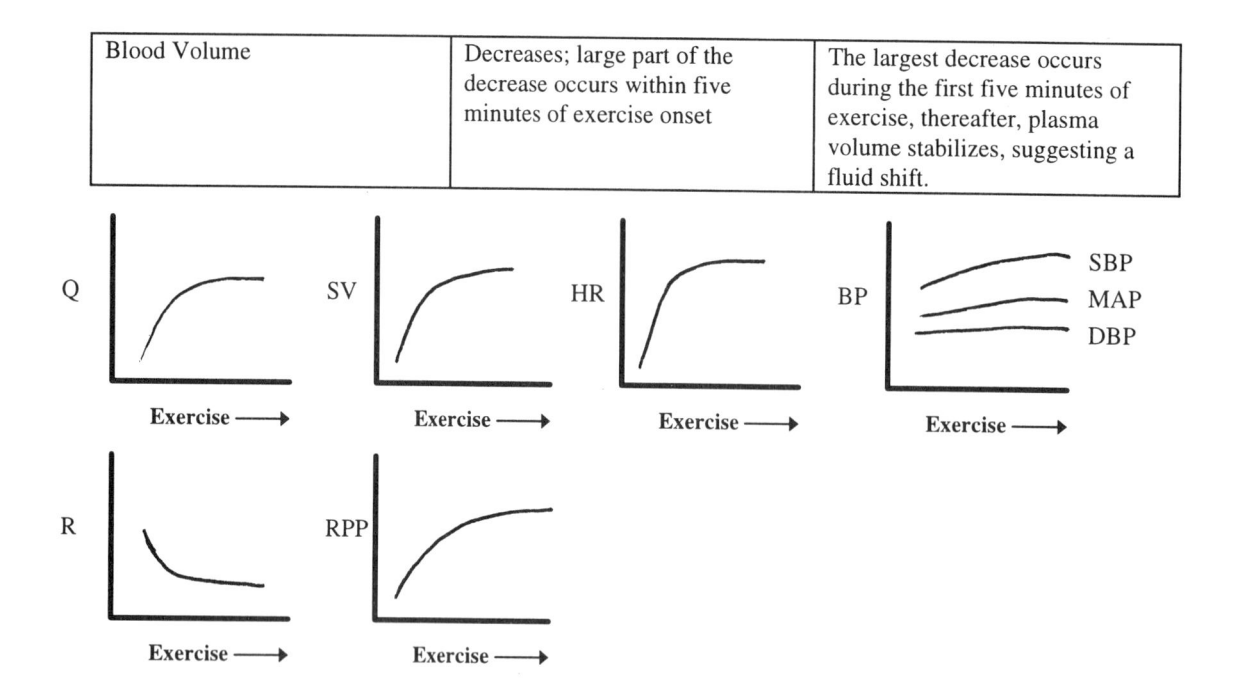

Blood Volume	Decreases; large part of the decrease occurs within five minutes of exercise onset	The largest decrease occurs during the first five minutes of exercise, thereafter, plasma volume stabilizes, suggesting a fluid shift.

Q [graph: rising curve leveling off] Exercise →   SV [graph: rising curve leveling off] Exercise →   HR [graph: rising curve leveling off] Exercise →   BP [graph: SBP, MAP, DBP] Exercise →

R [graph: decreasing curve] Exercise →   RPP [graph: rising curve leveling off] Exercise →

2. Graph and explain the pattern of response for which of the major cardiovascular variable during prolonged, heavy dynamic exercise. Explain the mechanisms responsible for each response.
Figure 5.4; table 5.1; pgs. 115-119.

Variable	Pattern of Response	Mechanism
Cardiac Output	Increase rapidly, levels off	Due to the increase in both stroke volume and heart rate
Stroke Volume	Increase rapidly, levels off ; drifts downward after 30 minutes of exercise	During the first 30 minutes of exercise the increase in SV is the result of an increased venous return (Frank-Starling response, increased contractility, activation of the sympathetic nervous system). If exercise continues beyond 30 minutes, the downward drift is SV is largely due to an attempt to redirect blood to the cutaneous vessels.
Heart Rate	Increase rapidly, levels off; drifts upward after 30 minutes of exercise	Related to the intensity of the exercise. The response is due to parasympathetic withdrawal and activation of sympathetic nervous system. After 30 minutes there may be an upward drift. The increase in HR is proportional to the decrease in SV. This drift is an attempt to compensate for the downward drift in SV to maintain cardiac output.

Systolic Blood Pressure	Increase rapidly, levels off ; drifts downward after 30 minutes of exercise	Reflects the increase in cardiac output.
Diastolic Blood Pressure	No change	
Mean Arterial Pressure	Increases initially; little drift	Due to increase in cardiac output, and is mediate by a large decrease in resistance.
Total Peripheral Resistance	Decreases rapidly, levels off; may drift downward after 30 minutes of exercise	Due to the vasodilation of the active muscles and cutaneous vessels to dissipate the heat produced..
Rate Pressure Product	Increase rapidly, levels off ; drifts upward after 30 minutes of exercise	Due to increases in both heart rate and SBP.

Q [graph vs Exercise] SV [graph vs Exercise] HR [graph vs Exercise] BP [graph vs Exercise] — SBP, MAP, DBP

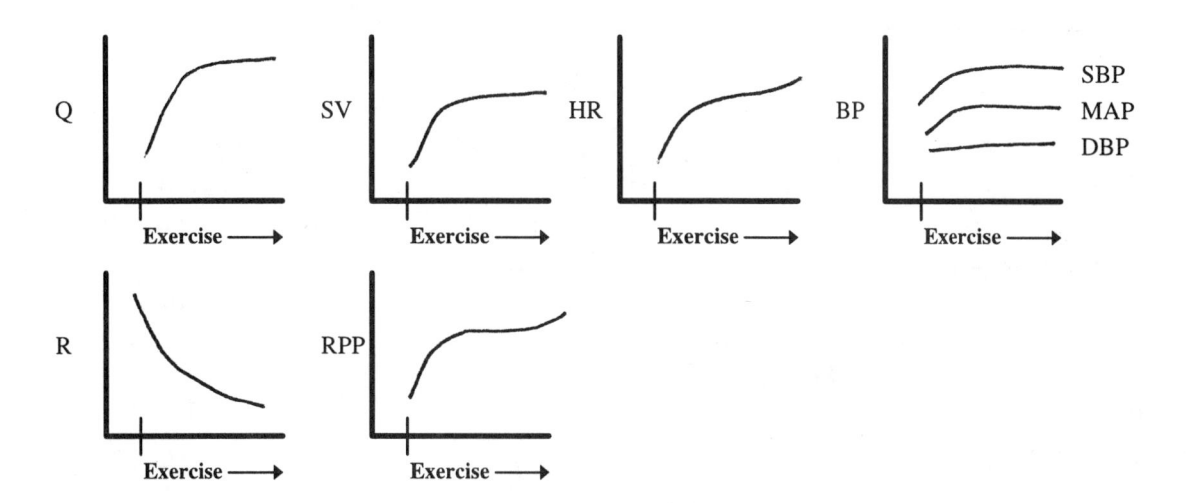

R [graph vs Exercise] RPP [graph vs Exercise]

3. Graph and explain the pattern of response for each of the major cardiovascular variables during incremental exercise to maximal. Explain the mechanisms responsible for each response.
Figure 5.7; Table 5.1; pgs. 119-121.

Variable	Pattern of Response	Mechanism
Cardiac Output	Rectilinear increase, plateau at max	Due to the increase in both stroke volume and heart rate, but with workloads greater than 40-50% VO_2max, the increase is achieved solely by an increase in HR
Stroke Volume	Increases, plateaus at approximately 40-50% VO_2 max	LVEDV increases because of the return of blood to the heart by the active muscle pump and the increased sympathetic outflow to the veins that results in venoconstriction. LVESV decreases because of augmented contractility of the heart.

Heart Rate	Rectilinear increase, plateau at max	Initially due to parasympathetic withdrawal and activation of sympathetic nervous system.
Systolic Blood Pressure	Rectilinear increase, plateau at max	Reflects the increase in cardiac output.
Diastolic Blood Pressure	No change	Due to balance of vasodilation in the vasculature of the active muscles and vasoconstriction in other vascular beds.
Mean Arterial Pressure	small rectilinear increase	Due to increase in cardiac output.
Total Peripheral Resistance	Decreases sharply, levels off	Due to the vasodilation of the active muscles and cutaneous vessels to dissipate the heat produced.
Rate Pressure Product	Rectilinear increase, plateau at max	Due to increases in both heart rate and SBP.

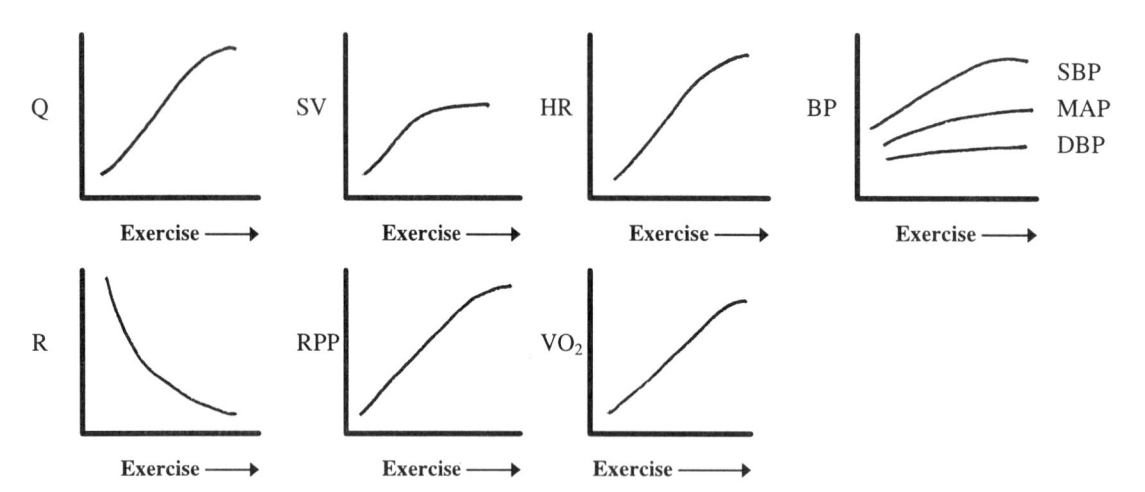

Q [graph] Exercise →   SV [graph] Exercise →   HR [graph] Exercise →   BP [graph, SBP/MAP/DBP] Exercise →

R [graph] Exercise →   RPP [graph] Exercise →   VO₂ [graph] Exercise →

4. Graph and explain the pattern of response for each of the major cardiovascular variables during static exercise. Explain the mechanisms responsible for each response. **Figure 5.17; Table 5.1; pgs. 131-134.**

Variable	Pattern of Response	Mechanism
Cardiac Output	Modest increase	Due to the increase in heart rate.
Stroke Volume	no change at low workloads; decreases at high workloads	Decrease in venous return (preload) due to high intrathoracic pressure and increase in blood pressure (afterload)
Heart Rate	Increases	Vagal withdraw and increase in sympathetic nerve activity.
Systolic Blood Pressure	Large increase	Pressor reflex stimulated by muscle mechano- and metaboreceptors
Diastolic Blood Pressure	Large increase	Pressor reflex stimulated by muscle mechano- and metaboreceptors

Mean Arterial Pressure	Large increase	Pressor reflex stimulated by muscle mechano- and metaboreceptors
Total Peripheral Resistance	Decreases modestly	Vasodilation is partially offset by mechanical constriction.
Rate Pressure Product	Large increase	Due to increases in both heart rate and SBP.

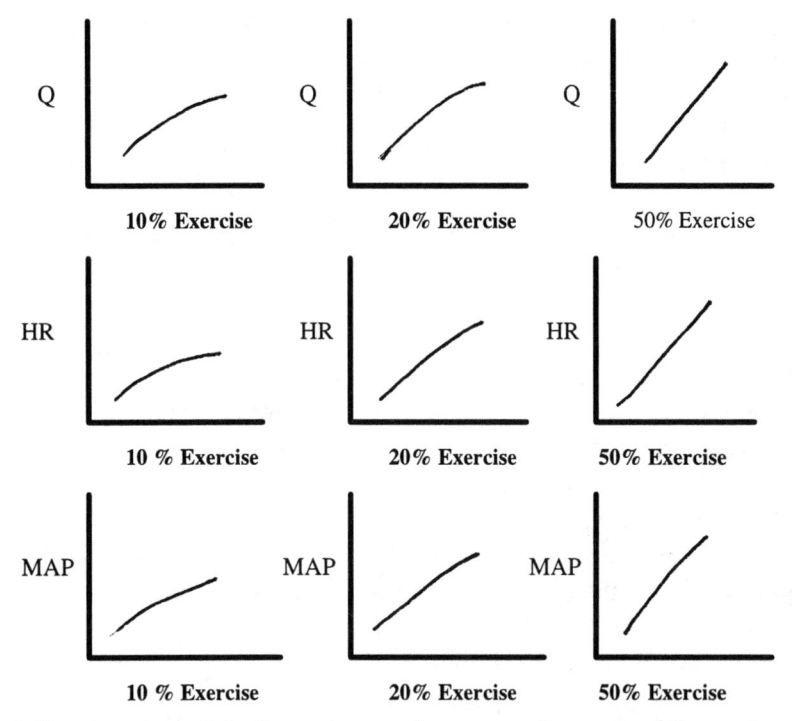

Q | 10% Exercise   Q | 20% Exercise   Q | 50% Exercise

HR | 10 % Exercise   HR | 20% Exercise   HR | 50% Exercise

MAP | 10 % Exercise   MAP | 20% Exercise   MAP | 50% Exercise

5. Graph and explain the patterns of response for each of the major cardiovascular variables during dynamic resistance exercise. Explain the mechanisms responsible for each response.

Pgs. 135-138

Variable	Pattern of Response	Mechanism
Cardiac Output	Modest increase	Due to the increase in heart rate.
Stroke Volume	little change, slight increase	
Heart Rate	Increase	Parasympathetic withdraw and increase in sympathetic nerve activity.
Systolic Blood Pressure	Increase	Due to increase in Cardiac Output, possibly response initiated by mechano- and metaboreceptors in muscle
Diastolic Blood Pressure	no change or increase	
Mean Arterial Pressure	Increase	Due to increase in Cardiac Output
Rate Pressure Product	Increase	Due to increases in both heart rate and SBP.

6. Discuss the change that occurs in total peripheral resistance during exercise, and explain its importance for blood flow and blood pressure. Why is resistance altered in older adults?

Pgs. 112-119, 130
Resistance decreases in all types of exercise due to vasodilation in active muscle in response to the need for increase blood flow to the active tissues. The decrease in resistance is important in keeping the mean arterial pressure from an exaggerate increase.
The higher resting resistance and smaller decrease in resistance during exercise that is reported in older adults is due to a loss of elasticity in the vasculature.

7. Describe the pressor response to static exercise, and explain the mechanisms by which blood pressure is elevated.

Pgs. 131-135
The pressor response is the exaggerated blood pressure response to static contraction. Static exercise increases metabolic demands to the active muscle, and high intramuscular tension results in mechanical constriction which impedes blood flow to the muscle. This results in a local build up of metabolic by products, which stimulates sensory nerve endings, leading to a pressor reflex, causing a rise in mean arterial pressure (Pressor Response). This increase in mean arterial pressure is substantially larger than dynamic exercise response requiring similar energy expenditure.

Chapter 5

CARDIOVASCULAR RESPONSE TO EXERCISE
Exam Questions

A. Multiple Choice

1. The difference in cardiovascular response between static and dynamic (aerobic) exercise is that:
   a. Static activity causes a smaller response in heart rate and blood pressure than does dynamic aerobic activity.
   b. Static activity causes a smaller response in heart rate and a larger rise in blood pressure than does dynamic aerobic activity.
   c. Static activity causes a larger response in heart rate and a smaller rise in blood pressure than does dynamic aerobic activity.
   d. Static activity causes a larger response in heart rate and blood pressure than does dynamic aerobic activity.

   Answer- b

2. A heart rate of approximately 180 b·min^{-1} is considered maximal because:
   a. the cardiac muscle cells are producing lactic acid in quantities that inhibit enzyme action.
   b. the upper limit of the speed of neural transmission through the cardiac conduction system has been reached.
   c. diastole has reached the lower limit of effective filling time.
   d. the myocardium cannot contract and relax any faster.

   Answer- c

3. Cardiovascular variables change most dramatically in response to short term submaximal dynamic exercise:
   a. during the first 3 minutes.
   b. during the first 30 seconds.
   c. in the last 3 minutes.
   d. None of these: the response involves continual change.

   Answer- b

4. Cardiovascular drift are changes in the cardiovascular variables that occur during:
   a. light, submaximal exercise.
   b. incremental to maximal exercise.
   c. prolonged, heavy submaximal exercise.
   d. none of the above

Answer- c

5. Cardiovascular drift:
   a. occurs during static exercise.
   b. is an irregular blood pressure.
   c. occurs during a heart attack.
   d. is influenced by fluid ingestion.

Answer- d

6. During dynamic exercise:
   a. HR does not change.
   b. blood volume decreases.
   c. SBP decreases or does not change.
   d. SBP and DBP both increase.

Answer- b

7. During dynamic aerobic exercise, blood is:
   a. shunted from the brain.
   b. shunted from the skin.
   c. shunted from the G.I. tract.
   d. shunted from the muscles.

Answer- c

8. At what percent VO_2 max does stroke volume reach a steady rate in normal healthy adults?
   a. 40-50%
   b. 10-20%
   c. 90-100%
   d. 60-70%

Answer- a

9. In comparing 30% MVC static contractions to a treadmill max, which value(s) is (are) lower during static exercise?
   a. Q
   b. SBP
   c. HR
   d. a & c
   e. b & c

Answer- d

10. During maximal incremental exercise, blood flow to the working muscles represents approximately _____% of the cardiac output?
    a. 65
    b. 70
    c. 85
    d. 98

Answer- c

B. Fill In the Blank

1. The changes observed in cardiovascular variables that occur during prolonged, heavy submaximal exercise without a change in workload is called _____ _____.

Answer- Cardiovascular drift

2. The rapid increase in both systolic pressure and diastolic pressure during static exercise is called the _____ _____.

Answer- Pressor response

3. An exercise that is performed at an intensity such that the energy expenditure during exercise is balanced with the energy required to perform that exercise is _____ _____ _____.

Answer- Steady state exercise

4. Forcibly exhaling against a closed glottis is called the _____ _____.

Answer- Valsalva maneuver

5. _____ _____ _____ _____ is a series of progressively increasing work intensities that continues until the individual can do no more.

Answer- Incremental exercise to maximum

CARDIORESPIRATORY TRAINING PRINCIPLES AND ADAPTATIONS
Outline

I. Introduction

II. Application of the Training Principles

   A. Specificity

   B. Overload

      1. Intensity

         a. Heart Rate Methods

         b. Oxygen Consumption/% VO_2max Methods

         c. Rating of Perceived Exertion Methods

      2. Duration

      3. Frequency

   C. Individualization

   D. Adaptation

   E. Progression

   F. Maintenance

   G. Retrogression/Plateau/Reversibility

   H. Warm-Up and Cool-Down

III. Cardiovascular Adaptations to Endurance Training
- A. Cardiac Dimensions (1a)
- B. Coronary Blood Flow (1b)
- C. Blood Volume (2)
- D. Cardiac Output (3a)
- E. Stroke Volume (3b)
- F. Heart Rate (3c)
- G. Maximal Oxygen Consumption (4)
- H. Blood Pressure (5)
- I. Total Peripheral Resistance (6)
- J. Muscle Blood Flow (7)
- K. Rate-Pressure Product (8)
- L. Sex Difference in Adaptation
- M. Adaptations in Children
- N. Adaptations in the Elderly

IV. Cardiovascular Adaptations to Dynamic Resistance Training
- A. Cardiac Dimensions
- B. Stroke Volume and Heart Rate
- C. Blood Pressure
- D. Maximal Oxygen Consumption

Chapter 6

CARDIORESPIRATORY TRAINING PRINCIPLES AND ADAPTATIONS
Suggested Laboratory Activities

1. Have students write a cardiovascular-respiratory training program and explain how each training principle is incorporated in it.

2. Have students write a periodization cycle showing variation in cardiovascular intensity and training volume.

3. Prepare a variety of cardiovascular-respiratory work-outs such as:
   - run 3 miles on the treadmill at a self-selected pace and grade
   - ride a cycle ergometer for 25 minutes at a self-selected cadence and load
   - stair step on a StairMaster or similar piece of equipment at a self-selected rate for 25 minutes

   Monitor heart rate and rate of perceived exertion. Have each student determine %HRmax and %HRR at which the workout was completed and indicate the classification of intensity according to Table 6.2, p. 146.

4. Compare and contrast the measured cardiovascular exercise responses of the highest trained endurance individual, the best trained dynamic resistance individual and an untrained individual in the class (same sex) at:
   - the same absolute submaximal workload (heart rate)
   - maximal work (heart rate and maximal oxygen consumption)

Chapter 6

CARDIORESPIRATORY TRAINING PRINCIPLES AND ADAPTATIONS
Review Questions

1. How is overload manipulated to bring about Cardiorespiratory adaptation?

    Pgs. 150-152
    Overload is manipulated to cause cardiovascular adaptations by using the FIT principle in which frequency, intensity, and duration are altered (increased or decreased) to help produce desired results.

2. Differentiate between central and peripheral cardiovascular adaptations.

    Pg. 144
    The central cardiovascular system is comprised of both the heart and oxygen-delivery components of the body. These responses are the same regardless of what the activity may be: running, skating, or cycling all produce the same response. Many modalities can have the same overall training benefit with regard to adaptation of the central cardiovascular system. Peripheral cardiovascular system refers to the oxygen extraction in the musculature. Peripheral adaptations are specific to the muscle that is exercised. To maximize peripheral adaptation, closely related activities which mimic the muscle action are needed.

3. Compare and contrast cardiac output, stroke volume, heart rate, and blood pressure adaptations to endurance training at rest and during submaximal and maximal exercise.

    Figure 6.7; Table 6.5; Pgs. 156-161
    Resting cardiac output (Q) is unchanged following a training program, although it is achieved by a larger stroke volume (SV) and a lower heart rate (HR). During absolute submaximal exercise, Q is decreased or is unchanged following an endurance training program.

Maximal Q is increased following training. Resting stroke volume is higher following a training program This is due to an increase in plasma volume, increased cardiac dimensions, increased venous return, and an enhanced ability of the ventricle to stretch and accommodate increased venous return. Enhanced ventricular filling (increase LVEDV) and emptying (decrease LVESV) both contribute to the augmented SV in trained athletes, although ventricular filling has greater influence. Resting HR is lower in trained individuals (bradycardia). The HR response to an absolute submaximal workload is lower following an endurance training program. Blood Pressure (BP) reports little or no change in arterial blood during rest, submaximal exercise, or during maximal exercise. However, since the amount of work done at maximal level can be increased, then the systolic BP may be higher at maximal exercise.

4. Discuss the impact of an individual's initial-fitness level on expected improvements in fitness and health related benefits.

   Figure 6.1; Pg. 152
   An individual's initial fitness level is inversely related to health-related benefits that can be expected from an aerobic exercise training program. The greatest improvements in both fitness and health benefits occur when very sedentary individuals begin a regular, low to moderate, endurance type exercise program. Health related benefits can be achieved with minimal increases in activity or fitness.

5. Describe the physiological benefits of a warm-up and a cool-down period.

   Pgs. 155-156
   The physiological benefits of a warm-up include: an increase blood flow (BF) to the active skeletal muscle, an increase in BF to the myocardium, an increase in the dissociation of oxyhemoglobin, earlier sweating (which is important for temperature regulation), and a possible reduction in the incidence of abnormal rhythms on the conduction system of the heart (arrhythmia) which can lead to abnormal heart function. The cool-down period is important as it prevents venous pooling and thus reduces the risk of fainting.

6. Explain the changes in blood volume that occur as a result of an endurance training program.

   Figure 6.6; Pg. 157
   Blood volume can increase by 20-25% in highly trained endurance athletes. This is primarily due to an increase in blood plasma volume.

This increase occurs quickly, with increases of 8-10% within the first week of exercise.

7. Compare and contrast cardiovascular adaptations to endurance and resistance training.

Pgs. 156-161, 165-166

Variable	Dynamic Endurance Exercise	Dynamic Resistance Exercise
Cardiac Dimensions	Increase in LV diameter due to enhanced LV filling (preload)	Increased LV wall and septal thickness due to the work the heart must do to overcome the high arterial pressure (afterload)
HR	Lower resting and submaximal HR, no change in HR max	Resting HR -lower or no change Submaximal HR- lower Maximal HR- no change
SV	Increase in resting, submaximal, and max SV.	?
Q	Unchanged at rest & submaximal exercise, increased Qmax	?
BP	No change	No documented effect
VO_2max	Increased	Little or no change

Cardiac Dimensions-Both dynamic endurance and resistance training programs can result in change in cardiac dimensions. Endurance training is associated with an increased LV diameter, which accommodates the enhanced LV filling (preload) associated with this type of training. On the other hand, resistance training leads to an enhanced LV and septal wall thickness due to the work the heart must do to overcome high arterial pressure (afterload) associated with this type of training.

Heart Rate- Endurance training results in a marked reduction in resting and submaximal HR. Resistance training may also cause a reduction in resting and submaximal HR, but not to the same extent. Neither type of training has a meaningful effect on maximal HR.

Q-There is little scientific evidence as to the effect of resistance training on SV or Q, but it is unlikely that resistance training would lead to the large increases seen in resting, submaximal, and maximal SV that are associated with endurance training.

Blood Pressure-When normotensive individuals follow appropriate training programs, there is no consistent evidence of changes in BP for either type of exercise training.

VO₂max- Endurance training results in appreciable gains in VO_2max (often above 15% improvement), whereas, resistance training results in little or no change in VO_2max.

Chapter 6

CARDIORESPIRATORY TRAINING PRINCIPLES AND ADAPTATIONS
Exam Questions

A. Multiple Choice

1. Exercise intensity can be prescribed by using:
   a. Heart rate, either as a percentage of maximal heart rate, or as a percentage of heart rate reserve
   b. Maximal oxygen consumption, using a percentage value
   c. Rate of perceived exertion, either on a scale of 6-20 or 0(1) -10
   d. a, b, and c are correct

   Answer- d

2. A 65 yr. old healthy but previously sedentary man has a resting heart rate of 84 b·min^{-1}. His target heart rate ranges for a moderate workout by the %HRmax and the %HRR techniques, respectively, are:
   a. 78-115 b·min^{-1}; 127-140 b·min^{-1}
   b. 93-123 b·min^{-1}; 120-137 b·min^{-1}
   c. 93-140 b·min^{-1}; 120-144 b·min^{-1}
   d. 116-140; b·min^{-1} 141-144 b·min^{-1}

   Answer- b

3. A warm-up period has the following beneficial effects on cardiovascular function:
   a. It increases blood flow to the active skeletal muscles and the myocardium.
   b. It loads to the early onset of sweating which is important for regulation of body temperature.
   c. It may reduce the incidence of abnormal rhythms in the conduction system of the heart.
   d. a, b, and c are correct

   Answer- d

4. When comparing the effects and benefits of specific modality versus cross-training, which of the statements are accurate?
   a. Many forms of aerobic endurance activity or modalities can have the same overall effect on central cardiovascular function and adaptation.
   b. Specific activity or closely related activities which mimic the muscle action of the primary sport are needed to maximize peripheral adaptations.
   c. Cross-training can be beneficial for injury rehabilitation, baseline or off-season conditioning, and as recovery from an intense workout.
   d. a, b, and c are correct

Answer- d

5. When designing an exercise program for an individual, it is important to remember that:
   a. In general, training less than 2 days per week does not lead to improvement in VO_2 max; training more than 4 days per week leads to diminishing returns, although some minor improvement will be seen.
   b. Exercise sessions of less than 20 continuous minutes have no beneficial health or fitness effects.
   c. Greater improvements in VO_2max are achieved if the exercise sessions are shorter (25-35 min) and the intensity higher ($\geq 90\%$) than if the sessions are longer (35-45 min) and the intensity lower (50-90%).
   d. a, b, and c are correct

Answer- a

6. In order to maintain VO_2max levels the most important factor in the exercise prescription is:
   a. frequency
   b. intensity
   c. duration
   d. initial fitness level

Answer- b

7. Given the following information
   Subject = Pat   44 yrs   RHR = 70 b·min^{-1} VO_2max = 48 ml·kg^{-1}·min^{-1}
   Which of the following speeds should be recommended for this individual for a moderate intensity workout according to ACSM Guidelines?
   a. 3.5 mi·hr^{-1} = 12.9 ml·kg^{-1}·min^{-1} walking
   b. 5 mi·hr^{-1} = 30.3 ml·kg^{-1}·min^{-1} running
   c. 6.5 mi·hr^{-1} = 38.3 ml·kg^{-1}·min^{-1} running
   d. 8 mi·hr^{-1} = 46.4 ml·kg^{-1}·min^{-1} running

Answer- b

8. For the individual in the question above, what should the suggested target heart rate range be?
    a. 123-148 b·min^{-1}
    b. 137-160 b·min^{-1}
    c. 111-150 b·min^{-1}
    d. 105-158 b·min^{-1}

Answer- a

9. Which factor is most important in maintaining VO$_2$max?
    a. frequency
    b. duration
    c. intensity
    d. recovery

Answer- c

10. Which of the following is not a benefit of warming up?
    a. it increases blood flow to active skeletal muscles
    b. it increases blood flow to the myocardium
    c. it increases the disassociation of hemoglobin
    d. it increases blood flow to the digestive system

Answer- d

11. The greatest differences between sedentary and trained individuals are seen in which variable:
    a. HR max
    b. SV
    c. SBP
    d. DBP

Answer- b

12. The development or maintenance of cardiovascular fitness by alternating between or concurrently training in two or more modalities is called:
    a. in-season training
    b. fitness training
    c. cross-training
    d. Bo-Jackson training

Answer- c

B. Fill in the Blank

1. _____ is called a reduction in resting heart rate.
Answer- Bradycardia

2. The ability to deliver and use oxygen under the demands of intensive, prolonged exercise or work is called _____ _____.
Answer- Cardiorespiratory fitness

3. _____ _____ are adaptations that occur in the heart and contribute to an increased ability to deliver oxygen.
Answer- Central cardiovascular adaptations

4. The development or maintenance of cardiovascular fitness by altering between or concurrently training in two or more modalities is called _____ _____.
Answer- Cross training

5. _____ _____ _____ are adaptations that occur in the vasculature or the muscles that contribute to an increased ability to extract oxygen
Answer- Peripheral cardiovascular adaptations

THERMOREGULATION

Outline

I. Introduction

II. Exercise in Environmental Extremes

III. Basic Concepts

    A. Measurement of Environmental Conditions

    B. Measurement of Body Temperature

    C. Thermal Balance

    D. Heat Exchange

    E. Heat Exchange During Exercise

IV. Exercise in the Heat: Cardiovascular Demands

    A. Factors Affecting Cardiovascular Response to Exercise in the Heat

        1. Acclimatization

        2. Fitness Level

        3. Body Composition

        4. Hydration Level

    B. Sex Differences in Exercise Response in Heat

    C. Exercise Response of Older Adults in the Heat

    D. Exercise Response of Children in the Heat

    E. Heat Illness
- 1. Heat Cramps
- 2. Heat Syncope
- 3. Heat Exhaustion
- 4. Heat Stroke
- 5. Prevention

V. Exercise in the Cold
- A. Cold-Induced Injuries
- B. Prevention
- C. Factors Influencing Cold Tolerance

Chapter 7

THERMOREGULATION
Suggested Laboratory Activities

1. Have students obtain weather conditions from a variety of location from the TV weather channel or the Internet. Ask them to identify conditions of concern and to describe precautions exercisers should follow in those circumstances.

2. Have students exercise at 40% VO_2max for 1 minute, 50% VO_2max for 1 minute, 60% VO_2max for 1 minute, and 70% VO_2max until the onset of sweating. Record the time at which sweating began. Correlate the time of onset of sweating with VO_2max.

3. Measure heart rate during 60 minutes of selected aerobic endurance activity at 75% VO_2max. Provide fluid replacement for one half of the class but not the other. Alternatively, use three groups: no fluid, water, and a commercial sports drink. Compare and contrast the responses.

Chapter 7

THERMOREGULATION

Review Questions

1. Diagram the thermal balance that is typically maintained at rest. Indicate how this balance is altered during exercise in hot and cold environments.

    Figure 7.2; table 7.4; Pgs. 175-178
    Thermal balance means heat gain equals heat loss. This balance is altered during exercise in both hot and cold conditions as muscle activity greatly increases heat production adding to the heat gain of the body. In hot conditions, sweating occurs to reduce the core body temperature. However, if the evaporative cooling is greatly impaired, and at the same time, heat loss via radiation, conduction, and convection is reduced in the heat, this may actually add to the heat gain of the body. In cold conditions, the body will lose heat as it travels down a thermal gradient. Protective clothing is needed to prevent/ reduce heat loss, or the body's temperature will decrease resulting in a decrease in performance and possible hypothermia.

2. Identify the factors that influence heat exchange and discuss how each factor facilitates or impedes the transfer of heat to and from the body.

    Pg. 177
    Factors that influence heat exchange include: thermal gradient, relative humidity, air movement, degree of direct sunlight, and clothing worn by the participant. Since the body is usually warmer than the environment and heat moves down a thermal gradient, more heat is lost on cooler days. On hot days the thermal gradient is less resulting in less heat loss. In fact, on extremely hot days the thermal gradient may cause head to be added to the body. High humidity decreases evaporative heat loss from the body since the air is already saturated with water. Relative humidity is the primary factor that determines the effectiveness of evaporative cooling. Air movement tends to increase convective heat loss from the skin to the environment; the more wind, the more heat is lost from the body. Direct sunlight adds to the radiant heat load of a person, whereas,

shade provides protection. Clothes protects against excessive heat loss during cold weather. However, clothing can also prevent the body from dissipating heat in hot weather. Dress with light colors on hot days to reflect sunlight.

3. Describe the cardiovascular responses to incremental exercise in a hot environment. Explain why these responses occur.

> **Figures 7.6, 7.7; Pgs. 178-180**
> Cardiovascular responses to incremental exercise includes an increase in cardiac output (Q). However, under hot conditions the maximal Q achieved is less than maximal Q under thermoneutral conditions. This is due to a lower maximal stroke volume (SVmax) and an unchanged maximal heart rate (HR). Exercise under hot conditions can not be performed for as long, resulting in a decrease in VO2max. Blood Flow (BF) also increases during exercise in the heat. However, skeletal muscle BF represents a smaller portion of total blood flow under hot conditions because skin BF is increased under hot conditions. Visceral BF is severely reduced during exercise under hot conditions in an effort to support the muscles with adequate BF and maintain blood pressure.

4. What is the importance of acclimatization? How much time is needed for acclimatization to occur?

> **Figure 7.8; Pgs. 180-181**
> Heat acclimatization is an adaptive change which occurs when an individual undergoes prolonged or repeated exposure to heat. It is important because it reduces the physiological strain associated with a hot environment. It has two effects: (1) it lowers HR and cardiovascular strain at a given level of exercise in the heat, and (2) it alters sweating patterns such that sweating begins earlier and continues at a higher rate for a given core temperature. Light to moderate exercise, for one to two hours per day can lead to acclimatization within a few days.

5. Explain the influence of hydration level on an individual's response to exercise in heat. What is necessary to maintain adequate hydration during exercise?

> **Pg. 182**
> Hydration is very important during exercise, especially under warmer conditions. Profuse sweating leads to large losses of total body water and a reduction in plasma volume if fluid is not replaced. This reduction of body fluid has a negative effect on performance and may lead to heat illness. However, if fluid is replaced, Q and

SV can be maintained throughout exercise. An individual should ingest 400-500 ml of water prior to activity and an additional 200-400 ml every 15-30 minutes during activity in warmer conditions. Thirst is an inadequate mechanism to maintain proper hydration.

6. Discuss the effects of fitness level and body composition on an individual's response to exercise in the heat.

   Pgs. 181-182
   The more fit an individual is, the better he or she can tolerate heat. Fit individuals have a lower resting core temperature, a larger plasma volume, an earlier onset of sweating, and a smaller decrease in plasma volume during exercise. Body composition also has an impact on thermoregulation as greater adiposity contributes to heat gain in two ways: (1) it interferes with the dissipation of heat since body fat insulates the core, and (2) body fat adds to the metabolic cost of weight bearing activity by adding weight to the body that must be removed. Heat illness is more common to overweight individuals.

7. Provide a definition, cause, and first aid for each of the following: heat cramps, heat syncope, heat exhaustion, and heatstroke.

   Pgs. 183-184
   Heat cramps are an acute disorder of brief, excruciating pain in the voluntary muscles of leg, arm, or abdomen. This is due to fluid/electrolyte imbalance and can be alleviated with water and a small amount of salt.
   Heat syncope is a temporary disorder characterized by circulatory failure due to pooling of blood in the peripheral veins and the subsequent decrease in ventricular filling which leads to a decrease in Q. It occurs most often in individuals in strenuous/unaccustomed exercise due to sudden rise in temperature and/or humidity. A cooler location should be sought and the individual should be allowed to rest in a recumbent position.
   Heat exhaustion is characterized by a rapid, weak pulse, fatigue, weakness, profuse sweating, psychological disorientation and fainting. Skin is often pale and clammy and body temperature is normal or moderately elevated. The individual should be moved to a cooler place, given fluids, and placed in a recumbent position.
   Heat stroke is a serious condition in which the skin and core temperature are elevated. Tachycardia, vomiting, diarrhea, hallucinations, and coma are symptoms of this condition. Heat stroke represents a failure of the thermoregulatory mechanisms.

First aid includes cooling the individual immediately (ice, fan, etc.). Medical attention is required. This is life-threatening.

8. Identify ways in which the likelihood of heat illness can be minimized.

   Pg. 184
   There are five general recommendations: (1) allow adequate time for acclimatization (10-14 days), (2) exercise during cooler parts of the day, (3) limit/defer exercise if heat stress index is in high risk zone, (4) hydrate properly prior to exercise and replace fluid loss during and after exercise (monitor daily weight changes), and (5) wear clothing that is light in color and loose fitting (large areas should be exposed for evaporation).

9. Explain the underlying cause of hypothermia and frostbite. Suggest ways in which these conditions can be prevented.

   Pgs, 185-186
   Hypothermia is a lowering of the core body temperature to the point that it affects its normal function. This occurs when heat loss exceeds that of heat production. Frostbite is a consequence of water crystallization within tissues which causes cellular dehydration and leads to tissue destruction. Prevention includes exercising judgment and wearing proper clothing outdoors in the cold. Layered clothing is best with windproof and water repellent outer garments. Avoid wearing cotton.

Chapter 7

THERMOREGULATION

Exam Questions

A. Multiple Choice

1. Environmental conditions that have the greatest affect on human thermoregulation are:
    a. ambient temperature, body weight, relative humidity
    b. ambient temperature, relative humidity, wind speed
    c. ambient temperature, cloud cover, barometric pressure
    d. ambient temperature, relative humidity, wind speed, body fat

Answer- b

2. Core temperature is normally maintained between:
    a. 31-34 °C
    b. 36-38 °C
    c. 39-42 °C
    d. 43-45 °C

Answer- b

3. Individual sweating rates are dependent upon:
    a. environmental conditions, ATP stores, fitness level, percent body fat, hydration status
    b. environmental conditions, relative humidity, iron status, percent body fat, hydration status
    c. environmental conditions, gender, percent body fat, degree of acclimatization, iron status
    d. environmental conditions, exercise intensity, fitness level, degree of acclimatization, hydration status

Answer- d

4. During exercise, heat production and heat transfer occur by the same mechanism as during resting conditions. However, metabolism may increase 15-20 times the resting rate and heat production may increase to a level greater than heat dissipation. Therefore, the body will:
   a. increase metabolic rate another 10% to increase heat dissipation.
   b. store heat and body temperature will increase
   c. increase vasodilation to the internal organs, such as the liver, to facilitate heat storage.
   d. decrease blood flow to the skin in an attempt to reduce sweating rate and maintain electrolyte balance.

Answer- b

5. Acclimatization to the heat involves which mechanisms?
   a. onset of sweating occurs earlier
   b. higher sweating rate
   c. increases in the partial pressure of oxygen at sea level that causes an increased unloading of oxygen during exercise
   d. a decreased heart rate at a given workload
   e. all of the above are correct
   f. a, b, and d are correct

Answer- f

6. Heat illness is more common in overweight individuals because the increased adiposity:
   a. causes an increase in blood viscosity thereby increasing stroke volume
   b. causes a decreased ability to dissipate heat
   c. increases the metabolic cost of the physical activity
   d. all of the above are correct
   e. b and c are correct

Answer- e

7. Voluntary dehydration is most likely caused by:
   a. a decrease in the ability of the thermohydration center to sense water loss
   b. a decrease in the water intake by the individual because stopping exercise to hydrate would decrease performance times
   c. thirst is not an adequate mechanism to tell an individual to hydrate
   d. an over powering coach

Answer- c

8. Which statement accurately describes the cardiovascular exercise response of an older individual in the heat:
   a. at higher workloads, there is a larger increase in cardiac output in an older individual when compared to a younger individual of a similar fitness level.
   b. at higher workloads, there is a smaller increase in cardiac output in an older individual when compared to a younger individual of a similar fitness level.
   c. at higher workloads, there is a larger increase in maximal heart rate of an older individual when compared to a younger individual of a similar fitness level.
   d. because heart rate max cannot increase, there is a compensatory increase in the DBP in an older individual when compared to a younger individual of a similar fitness level.

Answer- b

9. Place the following heat stress injuries in order from the least severe to the most severe. 1. Heat exhaustion 2. Heat cramps 3. Heat stroke 4. Heat syncope
   a. 1, 2, 3, 4
   b. 2, 4, 1, 3
   c. 2, 1, 3, 4
   d. 2, 4, 3, 1

Answer- b

10. Hypothermia is caused by which factors?
    a. core temperature $< 35°C$
    b. over dressing for environmental conditions
    c. a decreased heat production
    d. an increased heat loss
    e. all of the above are correct
    f. a, c, and d are correct

Answer- f

B. Fill in the Blank

1. _____ is the term to used to describe the adaptive changes that occur when an individual undergoes prolonged or repeated exposure to a stressful environment; the changes reduce the physiological strain produced by such an environment.
   Answer- Acclimatization

2. A spectrum of disorders that range in intensity and severity from mild cardiovascular and central nervous disorders to severe cell damage, including the brain, kidneys and liver is called _____ _____.
   Answer- Heat illness

3. The _____ _____ _____ is a scale used to determine the risk of heat stress from measures of ambient temperature and relative humidity.
   Answer- Heat stress index

4. _____ _____ is the moisture in the air relative to how much moisture, or water vapor that can be held by the air at any given ambient temperature.
Answer- Relative humidity

5. Exercise-induced dehydration that develops despite an individual's access to unlimited water is termed _____ _____.
Answer- Voluntary dehydration

Chapter 8

CARDIORESPIRATORY SYSTEM IN HEALTH AND DISEASE

Outline

I. Introduction

II. Physical Activity and Cardiovascular Risk Factors

    A. Major Modifiable Risk Factors

        1. Cholesterol-Lipid Fractions

        2. Cigarette Smoking

        3. Hypertension

        4. Physical Inactivity

    B. Contributing Modifiable Risk Factors

        1. Diabetes Mellitus

        2. Obesity

        3. Stress

    C. Selected Nontraditional Risk Factors

        1. Fibrinogen and Fibrinolytic Activity

III. Children and the Cardiovascular Risk Factors

    A. Cholesterol-Lipid Fractions

    B. Cigarette Smoking

    C. Hypertension

    D. Physical Inactivity

    E. Diabetes Mellitus

    F. Obesity

    G. Stress, Fibrinogen, and Fibrinolytic Activity

IV. Immune System, Exercise Training, and Illness

    A. Immune Response

    B. Effect of Exercise on Immune Response

        1. Innate Defense Mechanisms

        2. Adaptive Defense Mechanisms

    C. Hormonal Control of Immune Response to Exercise

    D. Training Adaptation

V. Selected Interactions of Exercise and Immune Function

    A. Exercise, the Immune System, and Upper Respiratory Tract Infection

    B. Exercise, the Immune System, and Cancer

    C. Exercise, the Immune System, and Aids

Chapter 8

CARDIORESPIRATORY SYSTEM SPECIAL APPLICATIONS
Suggested Laboratory Activities

1. Have each student evaluate his/her risk for cardiovascular disease. If modifiable risk factors are apparent, ask each student to give reasonable lifestyle changes that could be implemented.

2. Present one or more case study scenarios for individuals with a variety of symptoms (fever, sore throat, etc.). Ask students to determine if each individual should continue with normal exercise training or stop training.

Chapter 8

CARDIORESPIRATORY SYSTEM SPECIAL APPLICATIONS
Review Questions

1. Identify risk factors that cannot be changed, and discuss their relationship with cardiovascular disease.

    Table 8.1; Pgs. 191-195
    Risk factors that can not be changed include; age, race, heredity, and sex. Age is a risk factor for males over age 45 and females over age 55 or at the time of menopause without estrogen replacement. Blacks have a higher death rate from CVD than do whites. A family history of premature cardiovascular disease, diabetes mellitus, hypertension, and/or high cholesterol levels increase the risk of coronary heart disease.

2. Identify the major risk factors that can be modified, and discuss their relationship with cardiovascular disease.

    Table 8.1; Pgs. 195-197
    Cholesterol/Lipid Fractions -High levels of cholesterol (total cholesterol, TC) and LDL are associated with greater risk of CVD. High levels of HDL are inversely associated with CVD.
    Cigarette Smoking -The nicotine in cigarettes stimulates the sympathetic nervous system, causing an acute increase in HR and BP making the heart work harder. Carbon monoxide binds to the hemoglobin and reduces oxygen transport. Smoking injures the arterial wall lining and increases the level of circulating TC and decreases the amount of HDL. It also causes the platelets to adhere to each other, speeding up the rate of internal blood clotting and decreasing prostacyclin which is responsible for blood vessel dilation. As a result, it is life threatening, and causes CVD.
    Hypertension -Hypertension is a modifiable risk factor of CVD. Resultant high BP may injure the artery linings and begin the process of atherosclerosis.
    Physical Inactivity -Inactivity is associated with an increased risk of CVD. As only 10% of the American population participate in regular exercise, this represents a risk factor that could be positively

changed for 90% of the population. The greatest reduction in risk of CVD is realized when previously sedentary individuals initiate a modest exercise program.

3. Identify contributing factors that can be modified, and discuss their relationship with cardiovascular disease.

   Table 9.1; Pgs. 195-197
   Diabetes Mellitus -A metabolic disorder that increases a person's chance to have CVD. Diabetes is characterized by atherosclerosis, impaired myocardial contraction, and poor peripheral perfusion.
   Obesity-Obesity greatly increases the risk of CVD. Obesity is also associated in many of the other risk factors for CVD.
   Stress- The stress response is related to the psychological and physiological aspects of the individual. The relationship between stress and CVD is difficult to detail due to difficulties in defining and identifying different types of stress. Hostility does appear to be positively associated with incidence of CVD.

4. Identify nontraditional risk factors, and discuss their relationship with cardiovascular disease.

   Table 8.1
   Fibrinogen and Fibrinolytic Activity- Fibrinogen is a protein present in blood plasma that is converted into fibrin threads that form the basis of a blood clot. It increases blood platelet aggression and blood viscosity. An increased level of fibrinogen will increase the chances of having internal blood clotting, thereby increasing the risk of CVD. Fibrinolytic activity is the breakdown of fibrin clots, and thus, a high fibrinolytic activity reduces the chance of CVD.
   Apolipoproteins-Apo-A1 is the major apolipoprotein of HDL, and is thus associated with a reduction of CVD risk. A decrease in Apo-A1 and an increase in APO-B are related to levels of HDL and LDL. Apo-B is the major apolipoprotein of LDL and is thus inversely related to CVD risk. Exact levels of each are not agreed upon.
   Stress and fibrinogen and fibrinolytic Activity- Stress can cause an increase in resting heart rate, blood pressure, and respiratory rate, and a decrease in clotting time, and the breakdown of fat for fuel.

5. What is the relationship between each risk factor and exercise?

   Figure 8.4; Table 8.4; Pg. 195
   Exercise training increases the HDL fraction and may lower TC. As of yet, there is no direct relationship between smoking and exercise. Fewer people who exercise smoke regularly compared to the general

population. Exercise training brings about a reduction in SBP and DBP in hypertensive individuals. Regular training along with body fat/weight loss has been shown to restore near-normal glucose tolerance and increase insulin sensitivity in individuals with non-insulin dependent diabetes.

6. What is the importance of identifying cardiovascular disease risk factors in children?

   Pgs. 197-200
   It is important to identify CVD in young children because if it is identified at this time, it may be possible to reduce, delay or prevent the severity of CVD in their adulthood. Many of the risk factors identified track into adulthood.

7. Graphically present the two branches of the immune system, emphasizing how the two branches wok together.

   Figure 8.3, Pg. 201
   Many of the interaction between the two branches can be attributed to the central role of the macrophages. Macrophages destroy antigens via phagocytosis and play a central role in activation the adaptive immune system.

8. Describe the immune response to moderate aerobic exercise and to an exhaustive bout.

   Pgs. 202-204

	Moderate Exercise	Exhaustive Exercise
Innate Branch	increases number and activity of neutrophils	decreases number and activity of neutrophils for 24 hours
	increases number , percent, and activity of NK cells	decreases of NK cells activity
Adaptive Branch	increase the number of B and T cells (relative to intensity)	no change in T cells
	T cells increase	
	decrease in immumoglobulin (salivary)	

9. Differentiate between the training adaptations of the immune system to a moderate training program and to overtraining.

   Pg. 204

Moderate Training	Excessive Training
• enhanced NK cell activity	• decreased neutrophil killing capacity • decreased serum complement • decreased salivary immumoglobulin
immune function enhanced	immune function disturbed- may lead to illness

10. Describe the relationship between exercise and the incidence of URTI.

    Figure 8.4; Pgs. 204-206
    The relationship can be described as a "J-shaped" curve. Moderate exercise leads to a decrease in the incidence of URTI relative to a sedentary lifestyle, while overtraining is linked to a greater incidence of URTI than is seen with either a sedentary lifestyle or with moderate training.

11. Describe the relationship between physical activity levels and the risk of various cancers.

    Pg. 206
    Physical activity is associated with a lower prevalence and mortality rates for colon, breast, prostate, and lung cancers. The mechanisms responsible for the effects of exercise on cancer are unknown, but may be related to a better overall lifestyle, lower body fat, decreased stool transient time, and enhancement of antioxidant enzyme systems.

12. Describe the role of physical activity in the life of an individual infected with the HIV.

    Pgs. 206-207
    During the early stages of the disease, physical activity appears to be useful and may delay the progression of the disease. Exercise appears to be safe throughout the course of the disease.

Chapter 8

CARDIORESPIRATORY SYSTEM IN HEALTH AND DISEASE
Exam Questions

A. Multiple Choice

1. Given the following information, how many major modifiable risk factors for heart disease does this 55 yr. old male have?
   Total Cholesterol = 260 mg·dL^{-1} Non-Smoker
   Diabetic   Sedentary
   Blood Pressure   150/96mmHg   Mother died at 70 yrs from heart attack
   a. 1
   b. 2
   c. 3
   d. 4
   e. 5

Answer- c

2. Using the information given in question #1, how many <u>non-modifiable</u> risk factors does this person have?
   a. 1
   b. 2
   c. 3
   d. 4
   e. 5

Answer- b

3. The impact of exercise training on coronary heart disease risk factors include(s):
   a. an increase in HDL lipoproteins and a decrease in total cholesterol
   b. incomplete normalization of hypertension although both systolic and diastolic blood pressures will decrease somewhat
   c. direct elimination of cigarette smoking
   d. a, b, and c are correct
   e. a and b are correct

Answer- e

101

4. A total cholesterol level of 240 mg·dL^{-1} represents _____ times the risk of a measurement of 200 mg·dL^{-1}?
   a. 1
   b. 2
   c. 3
   d. 4

Answer- b

5. Which of the following are reactions in the body caused by cigarette smoking?
   a. stimulated sympathetic nervous system
   b. increased heart rate
   c. increased blood pressure
   d. reduced oxygen transport
   e. all of the above are correct.
   f. none of the above are correct.

Answer- e

6. As the result of aerobic exercise training
   a. there can be a 10 mmHg decrease in both the SBP and the DBP.
   b. there can be changes in blood pressure observed within 3 weeks after the onset of training.
   c. blood pressure may be reduced 1 to 9 hours post exercise.
   d. All of the above are true.
   e. None of the above are true.

Answer- d

7. The relationship between CHD and level of physical activity can be described as:
   a. proportional.
   b. direct.
   c. inverse.
   d. U shaped.

Answer- c

8. The most important element of training for deriving a *health benefit* from the activity is:
   a. duration.
   b. intensity.
   c. frequency.
   d. a, and b
   e. a and c
   f. a, b, and c

Answer- e

9. Tim has been training for the spring season of rowing. He has been working out 3-4 hours per day, 7 days per week. He has been maintaining this particular schedule for the last 3 months. He recently became very sick. The sickness may be related to his apparent 'overtraining' and caused by:
   a. a depressed level of NK cells, which increased his vulnerability to infection.
   b. an increased level of NK cells, that in turn decreased his immune defense mechanism.
   c. a depressed level of T cells, that lasted for the first 30 minutes following exercise, and then increased above normal values.
   d. an increased level of NK cells, that lasted for the first 30 minutes following each day of exercise.

Answer- a

10. A _____ shaped model has been used to describe the relationship between physical activity and the risk of URTI:
   a. S
   b. inverted U
   c. U
   d. J

Answer- d

B. Fill in the Blank

1. An aspect of personal behavior or lifestyle, environmental exposure, or an inherited characteristic that has been shown by epidemiological evidence to predispose an individual to the development of a specific disease is called _____ _____.

2. Answer-Risk factor

3. _____ is a derived fat that is essential for the body. It can be synthesized in the liver and ingested from animal sources from the diet.
Answer- Cholesterol

4. _____ is a specific type of protein whose function is to transport fat in the bloodstream.
Answer- Apolopoprotein

5. A lipoprotein in blood plasma composed of protein, a small portion of triglyceride, and a large portion of cholesterol whose purpose is to transport cholesterol to the cells is _____ _____ _____.
Answer- Low density lipoprotein (LDL)

6. _____ is a term that describes the natural aging changes that occur in blood vessels-namely thickening of the walls, loss of elastic connective tissue, increase in calcium content, and increase in diameter.
Answer- Arteriosclerosis

7. _____ is a term that describes a pathological process that results in the buildup of plaque inside the blood vessels.
Answer- Atherosclerosis

8. A lipoprotein in blood plasma composed of protein and cholesterol or triglyceride whose purpose is to transport cholesterol from the tissues to the liver is called _____ _____ _____.
Answer- High-density lipoprotein (HDL)

9. _____ _____ _____ is a behavior that is characterized by hard-driving competitiveness, time urgency, haste, impatience; a workaholic lifestyle; and hostility.
Answer- Type A behavior pattern (TABP)

10. _____ _____ _____ is associated with characteristics or relaxation without guilt and no sense of urgency.
Answer- Type B behavior pattern (TBBP)

11. _____ is a protein present in blood plasma that, under the proper physiological circumstances, is converted into fibrin threads that form the basis of a blood clot.
Answer- Fibrinogen

12. The breakdown of the fibrin clots is called _____ _____.
Answer- Fibrinolytic activity

13. _____ is a personal phenomenon in which a characteristic is maintained, in terms of relative rank, over a long span or even a lifetime.
Answer- Tracking

Chapter 9

ENERGY PRODUCTION

Outline

I. Introduction

II. Cellular Respiration

   A. Carbohydrate Metabolism

      1. Stage I: Glycolysis Overview

         a. Oxidation-Reduction

         b. The Steps of Stage I

         c. Mitochondria

      2. Stage II: Formation of Acetyl Coenzyme A

      3. Stage III: Krebs Cycle

      4. Stage IV: Electron Transport and Oxidative Phosphorylation

      5. ATP Production from Carbohydrate

   B. Fat Metabolism

      1. Beta Oxidation

      2. ATP Production from Fatty Acids

      3. Ketone Bodies and Ketosis

   C. Protein Metabolism

      1. Transamination and Oxidative Deamination

      2. ATP Production from Amino Acids

III. The Regulation of Cellular Respiration and ATP Production

   A. Intracellular

   B. Extracellular

   C. Neurohormonal Coordination

IV. Fuel Utilization at Rest and During Exercise

Chapter 9

ENERGY PRODUCTION
Suggested Laboratory Activities

---

1. Describe a variety of exercise work-outs. Have students determine the relative degree of fuel utilization for muscle glycogen, liver glycogen, blood borne glucose, free fatty acids, and amino acids in each based on Table 9.5, p. 239.

Chapter 9

ENERGY PRODUCTION
Review Questions

1. Distinguish between anabolism and catabolism. Is cellular respiration anabolic or catabolic?

   Pgs. 213-214
   Anabolism- energy transformation is which small molecules are combined to make a larger one resulting in the build up of tissues; requires the utilization of ATP energy.
   Catabolism- energy transformation in which large molecules are broken down into smaller ones and energy is produced; the production of ATP from the breakdown of carbohydrate, fat, or protein.

2. Name and briefly summarize the four steps of carbohydrate metabolism.

   Figures 9.4, 9.5, 9.7, 9.8, 9.9, 9.11; Pgs. 215-226
   The four stages of carbohydrate metabolism are:
   I. Glycolysis
   - begins with glucose or glycogen
   - consists of 10 (aerobic) or 11 (anaerobic) steps
   - ends with pyruvic acid (aerobic) or lactic acid (anaerobic)
   - produces 2 (glucose) or 3 (glycogen) ATP as net gain by substrate level phosphorylation and 2 NADH + H^+
   II. Formation of Acetyl CoA
   - begins with pyruvic acid
   - consists of 2 steps
   - ends with acetyl CoA
   - produces 2 NADH + H^+
   III. Krebs Cycle
   - begins with acetyl CoA combining oxoloacetate
   - consists of 8 steps
   - ends with Oxaloacetate
   - produces 2 ATP directly by substrate level phosphorylation, 6 NADH + H^+ and 2 $FADH_2$
   IV. Electron Transport and Oxidative Phosphorylaton

- begins with the release of the hydrogen ions (H⁺) and electrons from NAD⁺ and FAD
- proceeds as a series of chemical reactions that shuttles the electrons along the respiratory chain cytochromes. The final electron acceptor is oxygen. The H+ are transported into the intermembrane space creating an electro-chemical gradient and current. This electrical energy synthesizes ATP from ADP + P₂.
- 32 ATP (skeletal muscle) or 34 ATP (cardiac muscle) are produced by oxidative phosphorylation.

3. Explain how a count of 36 ATP is achieved if the fuel substrate is glucose in skeletal muscle. Why is the ATP count from carbohydrate sometimes 37, 38, or 39 in stead of 36?

   Table 9.1; Pgs. 225-226
   A count of 36 ATP is achieved if the fuel substrate is glucose in skeletal muscle by:
   - 2 ATP from direct substrate level phosphorylation; glycolysis
   - 4 ATP from NADH + H⁺ ─ FADH₂; glycolysis
   - 6 ATP from 2 NADH + H⁺; stage II
   - 2 ATP from substrate level phosphorylation; Krebs cycle
   - 22 ATP from FADH₂ + NADH + H⁺; Krebs cycle; oxidative phosphorylation

Tissue	Substrate	ATP Yield
skeletal muscle	glucose	36
	glycogen	37
cardiac muscle	glucose	38
	glycogen	39

   Glucose always produces 1 less ATP than glycogen because glycogen enters after step 1 where 1 ATP is used, thereby yielding a net gain of 3, not 2 ATP, for glycolysis. Skeletal muscle always produces 2 less ATP than cardiac muscle because the hydrogens are transferred from NAD⁺ to FAD in the glycerol-phosphate shuttle (skeletal muscle) but continue to be carried by NAD⁺ in the malate-aspartate shuttle (cardiac muscle) when the hydrogens from glycolysis cross the mitochondria membrane.

4. Why is beta oxidation necessary before fat can be used as an energy substrate? Describe what occurs during beta oxidation.

> **Figure 9.14; Pgs. 230-231**
> Beta oxidation is necessary to reduce the fat from a 14-24 carbon unit (that it typically is) to a 2 carbon unit. This 2 carbon unit can be converted to acetyl CoA, enter the Krebs cycle, and subsequently undergo Electron Transport and Oxidative Phosphorylation.
> In beta oxidation, the fatty acid is first activated by the break down of ATP to AMP. Concurrently, coenzyme A is added. Hydrogens are removed with one pair being picked up by FAD and the other by NAD^+. The bond is broken between the alpha carbon (C_2) and the beta carbon (C_3), resulting in the removal of two carbons ($C_1 + C_2$). These 2 carbons are then used to form acetyl coenzyme A. This process is repeated for all but the last pair of carbons since the last pair form acetyl CoA itself.

5. State how the calculation is completed to determine the number of ATP produced from fatty acids. Complete an example using a fat having 24 carbons. Only even numbers can be used..

> **Pg. 231**
> a. *n/2-1 = 24/2-1 = 11 times through beta oxidation*
> b. each cycle produces 1 FADH2 and 1 NADH + H+ which in turn produce 5 ATP *11 x 5 = 55 ATP*
> c. each time through beta oxidation (11) plus the last step (1) produces acetyl CoA. Each acetyl CoA yields 1 ATP, 3 NADH, and 1 FADH₂ in the Krebs cycle for a net gain of 12 ATP for each acetyl CoA. *12 x 12 = 144 ATP*
> d. *144 ATP + 55 ATP = 199 ATP minus 2 ATP used in activation = 197 ATP from a 24 carbon fat.*

6. Name and describe the process that amino acids must undergo before being used as a fuel substrate. Why is this process necessary?

> **Figure 9.2; Pgs. 232-233**
> Amino acids must undergo transamination or oxidative deamination before being used as a fuel. This is necessary because all amino acids contain an amino group (NH_2) which must be removed before it can enter the Krebs Cycle. Transamination simply involves the transfer of the NH_2 amino group from an amino acid to a keto acid, resulting in a new amino acid and different keto acid. Deamination is the removal of the amino group which produces ammonia and an keto acid.

7. Identify the locations in the metabolic pathways where amino acids may enter. How does the ATP count differ between these locations?

> **Figure 9.2; Pg. 233**
> Amino acids can enter the metabolic pathways as pyruvic acid, as acetyl CoA, or in several locations in the Krebs cycle. The latter are converted to pyruvate before being used. If the amino acid is used as pyruvate 15 ATP are produced; if the amino acid enters as acetyl CoA, 12 ATP are produced.

8. Why is acetyl coenzyme A called the universal common intermediate?

> **Figure 9.2; Pg. 215**
> Acetyl CoA is called the universal common intermediate because all foodstuff whether it goes through glycolysis, beta oxidation, or transamination/oxidative deamination can and does form acetyl CoA before entering the Krebs cycle and ET/OP.

9. Why would the breath of someone suffering from anorexia nervosa smell sweet?

> **Pgs. 231-232**
> When the supply of glucose is inadequate, oxaloacetate must be converted into glucose, and because it is no longer available to bind to acetyl CoA, the acetyl CoA from the fatty acid is converted into 3 forms of ketones (acetoacetic acid, beta-hydroxybutyric acid, and acetone). It is the acetone that gives the sweet fruity smell in anorexic individuals who typically have inadequate diets, hence insufficient glucose supplies.

10. Describe the role of enzymes in the metabolic pathways. Identify the rate limiting enzymes in stages I, III, and IV of carbohydrate metabolism. How are enzymes regulated?

> **Pgs. 217-218**
> Enzymes catalyze each step in the metabolic pathways. Enzymes speed up the rate of a chemical reaction without themselves being altered by the reaction.
> Rate limiting enzymes:
> - Stage I   Phosphofructokinase (PFK)
> - Stage II Isocitrate dehydrogenase (ICD)
> - Stage III Cytochrome oxidase
>
> Enzymes are regulated by modulators. Positive modulators stimulate the production of ATP (positive feedback), negative modulators inhibit the production of ATP (negative feedback).

Positive Modulators	Negative Modulators
ADP	ATP
AMP	CP
P_i 2	Citrate
increase in pH	FFA
	decrease in pH

11. What are the goals of metabolic regulation during exercise? How are these goals achieved by the interaction of the sympathetic nervous system and the hormonal system?

>**Figure 9.16; Table 9.3; Pgs. 234-237**
>The goals of metabolic regulation during exercise are:
>a. to provide sufficient fuel for ATP production to meet the energy demands.
>b. to maintain blood glucose levels at near resting values because the brain and nervous system must have glucose as a fuel.
>
>These goals are achieved by the coordinated actions of the sympathetic nervous system and the endocrine system. The catecholamines (epinephrine and norepinephrine) and glucagon are released in a matter of seconds to minutes and insulin is suppressed. The result is a decrease in glucose uptake by nonactive cells, a decrease in glycogenesis and lipogenesis and an increase in glycogenolysis, glyconeogenesis and lipolysis. If the exercise continues for a long period of time, growth hormone and cortisol reinforce all the reduction in glycogenesis (bringing about an increase in glycogen formation in a further attempt to conserve carbohydrate). They also make protein available as a fuel source. Thyroxine potentiates the effect of the other hormones.

1. Compare the relative availability and use of carbohydrate, fat, and protein fuel substrates on the basis of intensity and duration of exercise.

    Tables 9.4, 9.5, 9.6; Pgs. 237-239
    The relative availability of the energy substrates is as follows:
    - Fat- highest by far
    - Protein- medium, but not desirable to use muscle mass as fuel
    - Carbohydrate- low

    The relative use of the energy substrates is as follows:

	Exercise Continuum- Dynamic Rhythmical Exercise			
	Low Intensity Long Duration			High Intensity Short Duration
Fat	High	Medium		Low
CHO	Low/Medium	Medium		High
Protein	Low			Negligible

	Rest	Static & very intense dynamic exercise
Fat	High	Negligible
CHO	High/Medium	High
Protein	Low	Negligible

112

Chapter 9

ENERGY PRODUCTION
Exam Questions

A. Multiple Choice

1. The advantage of metabolism proceeding through Glycolysis, the Krebs Cycle and Electron Transport/Oxidative Phosphorylation by a series of steps as opposed to one or two primary changes is that:
    a. less energy is converted to carbon dioxide this way.
    b. less oxygen is used to produce ATP.
    c. energy is released gradually and less is lost as heat averting tissue damage.
    d. energy production is more finely tuned to energy utilization.

Answer- c

2. The difference between aerobic or slow glycolysis and anaerobic or fast glycolysis is that:
    a. glycogen predominates as the fuel for slow glycolysis, and glucose predominates as the fuel of fast glycolysis.
    b. aerobic glycolysis yields 3 ATP, while anaerobic glycolysis yields only 2 ATP.
    c. Pyruvic acid (pyruvate) is the end product of aerobic glycolysis, while lactic acid (Lactate) is the end product of anaerobic glycolysis.
    d. FAD is the hydrogen carrier in anaerobic glycolysis, but NAD + is the hydrogen carrier in aerobic glycolysis.

Answer- c

3. Fat is an excellent storage fuel because:
    a. it is more energy dense (kcal·g^{-1}) than either carbohydrate or protein (4 kcal·g^{-1}).
    b. it is stored dry (whereas each gram of glycogen is stored with 2.7 g H$_2$0) thus the energy content is not diluted and bulk is saved.
    c. fat stores can last as long as 47 days of rest or 87 hours of running, whereas glycogen stores can be depleted in as little as 1 day of rest and 2 hours of heavy exercise.
    d. a, b, and c are correct

Answer- d

4. The primary function of the Krebs cycle is:
   a. to complete the oxidation of acetyl CoA derived from carbohydrates, fats, and proteins and from NADH + H$^+$ and FADH$_2$.
   b. to produce ATP via substrate-level phosphorylation.
   c. to prime glycolysis for the production of ATP.
   d. to produce H$_2$0 and ATP.

Answer- a

5. The name of the process and what it accomplishes before fatty acids can be used as a fuel are:
   a. transamination/oxidative-deamination, the removal of nitrogen and addition of phosphate.
   b. Beta oxidation, breaking off of pairs of carbons to form acetyl CoA.
   c. lipogenesis, anabolized into triglyceride.
   d. Gluconeogensis, converted to carbohydrate.

Answer- b

6. The principle function of glycolysis is to:
   a. degrade glucose or glycogen into pyruvic acid or lactic acid and produce ATP.
   b. form NADH + H$^+$ and FADH$_2$.
   c. degrade lactic acid to pyruvic acid.
   d. generate high-energy compounds such as GTP.

Answer- a

7. Once the reaction ATP 6 ADP + P$_i$ + Energy has occurred, ATP can be regenerated from ATP by:
   a. aerobic cellular respiration in the mitochondria.
   b. anaerobic cellular respiration in the mitochondria.
   c. interaction with CP (PC) in the cell cytoplasm.
   d. a, b, and c are correct
   e. a and c are correct

Answer- e

8. The name of the process and what it accomplishes before protein (amino acids) can be used as a fuel are:
   a. transamination/deamination, the removal of nitrogen in the form of ammonia.
   b. Beta oxidation, breaking off pairs of carbons to form acetyl CoA.
   c. transamination/deamination, the removal of nitrogen and addition of phosphate.
   d. gluconeogenesis, converted to carbohydrate.

Answer- a

9. Match the primary rate limiting enzyme from Column II with the stage of metabolism that it regulates in Column I.

COLUMN I
1. Stage I (Glycolysis)
2. Stage III (Krebs Cycle)
3. Stage IV (ET/OP)

COLUMN II
A. Cytochrome oxidase
B. Hexokinase
C. Phosphofructokinase
D. Pyruvate dehydrogenase
E. Isocitrate dehydrogenase

a. 1 = C; 2 = E; 3 = A
b. 1 = B; 2 = D; 3 = C
c. 1 = D; 2 = C; 3 = A
d. 1 = C; 2 = D; 3 = E

Answer- a

10. In Stage IV (Electron Transport/Oxidative Phosphorylation), ATP can be produced at 3 ball and stalk sites. These are located:
   a. between cytochromes b and c_1; c_1 and c; a and a_3.
   b. between coenzyme Q and cytochrome b; cytochromes b and c_1 and; cytochromes c and a.
   c. between Flavoprotein 1 and Coenzyme Q; cytochromes b and c_1 and cytochromes a and a_3.
   d. between Flavoproteins 1 and 2; between cytochromes c_1 and c and; a and a_3.

Answer- c

11. Match the location where the process takes place from Column II with the stage of Metabolism in Column I. (4 pts.)

COLUMN I
1. Stage I (Glycolysis)
2. Stage II
3. Stage II (Krebs Cycle)
4. Stage IV (ET/OP)

COLUMN II
A. inner mitochondrial membrane
B. mitochondrial matrix
C. capillary
D. cell membrane
E. cytoplasm

a. 1 = C; 2 = E; 3 = B; 4 = A
b. 1 = E; 2 = B; 3 = B; 4 = A
c. 1 = D; 2 = E; 3 = B; 4 = A
d. 1 = E; 2 = A; 3 = B; 4 = B

Answer- b

12. Carbohydrate is often called the preferred fuel of the body because:
    a. it is the only fuel substrate that can be used by certain tissues such as nerves and the brain.
    b. it is the only food nutrient that can be used to produce energy anaerobically.
    c. carbohydrate requires more oxygen to be metabolized than fat or protein.
    d. a and b are correct

Answer- d

13. The main benefit of glycolysis, beta oxidation, and oxidative deamination/transamination is that:
    a. they prepare carbohydrate, fat and protein to enter the common pathways of the Krebs Cycle, electron transport and oxidative phosphorylation.
    b. they each provide ATP anaerobically in the cell cytoplasm for quick energy needs.
    c. the CO_2 produced can easily be buffered by the HCO_3 - present without impacting pH.
    d. a, b, and c are correct

Answer- a

14. The difference in producing ATP by substrate level phosphorylation and oxidative phosphorylation is that:
    a. in substrate level phosphorylation, the phosphate is added to the food nutrient before it is catabolized in any fashion. In oxidative phosphylation, the fuel nutrient has first been broken down into acetyl CoA.
    b. in substrate level phosphorylation, the phosphate is transferred directly from the phosphorylated intermediates to ADP without any oxidation occurring.
    c. in oxidative phosphorylation, oxygen is converted to carbon dioxide when the phosphate is added. In substrate level phosphorylation, oxygen remains unchanged.
    d. a, b, and c are correct

Answer- b

15. Metabolism
    a. is the creation of energy to build tissues in the body.
    b. is the breakdown of foodstuffs so that energy is available to do work.
    c. is the total of all energy transformations that occur in the body.
    d. does not follow the *first law of thermodynamics*, which states that energy is neither created nor destroyed, but only changed in form.

Answer- c

16. ATP
    a. is cellular energy
    b. is adenosine triphosphate
    c. is a high-energy molecule
    d. all of the above

Answer- d

17. Complete the following reaction: ADP + P$_i$
    a. + work $\longrightarrow$ ATP
    b. + energy $\longrightarrow$ ATP
    c. + P $\longrightarrow$ ATP
    d. + ADP $\longrightarrow$ ATP

Answer- b

18. Acetyl Coenzyme A (acetyl CoA) is the central converting substance in the metabolism of
    a. fat
    b. protein
    c. CHO
    d. CHO and fat
    e. a, b, and c

Answer- e

19. Glycolysis occurs is the _____ of the cell.
    a. cristae
    b. mitochondria
    c. cytoplasm
    d. matrix

Answer- c

20. The two NADH + H$^+$ that are produced during glycolysis must use a shuttle system to enter the mitochondrial membrane. The two shuttle systems that operate for this purpose are:
    a. NADH shuttle system, and FADH$_2$ shuttle system
    b. malate-aspartate and glycerol-phosphate shuttle
    c. malate-aspartate and NADH shuttle
    d. glycerol-phosphate, and NADH shuttle

Answer- b

B.   Fill in the Blank

1. _____ is the total of all energy transformations that occur in the body.
   Answer- Metabolism

2. _____ is stored chemical energy that links the energy-yielding and energy requiring functions within all cells.
   Answer- Adenosine Triphosphate

3. A chemical process in which a substance is split into simpler compounds by the addition of water is termed _____.
   Answer- Hydrolysis

4. _____ are linked chemical processes in which a change in one substance is accompanied by a change in another.
   Answer- Coupled Reactions

5. The process by which cells transfer energy from food to ATP in a stepwise series of reactions is _____ _____
   Answer- Cellular Respiration

6. In the absence of, not requiring, or utilizing oxygen is _____.
   Answer- Anaerobic

7. A substance acted upon by an enzyme is a _____.
   Answer- Substrate,

8. _____ is a stored form of carbohydrate
   Answer- Glycogen,

9. The process by which stored glycogen is broken down (hydrolyzed) to provide glucose is _____.
   Answer- Glycogenolysis

10. The _____ _____ is a sequence of enzyme-mediated chemical reactions resulting in a specified product.
    Answer- Metabolic Pathway,

11. The energy pathway responsible for the initial catabolism of glucose in a 10- or 11-step process that begins with glucose or glycogen and ends with the production of pyruvate (aerobic glycolysis) or lactate (anaerobic glycolysis) is _____.
    Answer- Glycolysis

12. An _____ is defined by a protein that accelerated the speed of a chemical reaction without itself being changed by the reaction.
    Answer- Enzyme,

13. The transfer of P_i directly from phosphorylated intermediate or substrates to ADP without any oxidation occurring is _____ _____ _____.
Answer- Substrate-Level Phosphorylation

14. _____ is a gain of electrons.
Answer- Oxidation

15. _____ is a loss of electrons.
Answer- Reduction

16. _____ and _____ are hydrogen carriers in cellular respiration.
Answer- Nicotinamide Adenine Dinucleotide and Flavin Adenine Dinucleotide

17. The _____ are cell organelles in which the Krebs cycle, electron transport, and oxidative phosphorylation take place.
Answer- Mitochondria

18. _____ are nonprotein substances derived from a vitamin that activates an enzyme.
Answer- Coenzyme

19. A series of eight chemical reactions that begins and ends with the same substance; energy is liberated for direct substrate phosphorylation of ATP from ADP and P_i; carbon dioxide is formed and hydrogen atoms removed and carried by NAD and FAD to the electron transport system; does not directly utilize oxygen but requires its presence is called the _____ _____.
Answer- Krebs Cycle

20. The _____ _____ _____ is the final metabolic pathway; it proceeds as a series of chemical reactions in the mitochondria that transfer electrons from the hydrogen atom carriers NAD and FAD to oxygen; water is formed as a by-product; the electrochemical energy released by the hydrogen ions is coupled to the formation of ATP from ADP and P_i.
Answer- Electron Transport System

21. _____ _____ is the process in which NADH + H$^+$ and FADH$_2$ are oxidized in the electron transport system and the energy released is used to synthesize ATP from ADP and P_i.
Answer- Oxidative Phosphorylation

22. A cyclic series of steps that breaks off successive pairs of carbon atoms from FFA, which are then used to form acetyl CoA is called _____ _____.
Answer- Beta Oxidation

23. The transfer of the NH₂ amino group from an amino acid to a keto acid is _____.
Answer- Transamination

24. _____ is a term to describe the creation of glucose in the liver from noncarbohydrate sources, particularly glycerol, lactate or pyruvate, and alanine.
Answer- Gluconeogenesis

Chapter 10

ANAEROBIC METABOLISM DURING EXERCISE
Outline

I. The Energy Continuum

II. Measurement of Anaerobic Metabolism

    A. Laboratory Procedures

        1. ATP-PC and Lactate

        2. Tests of Anaerobic Power and Capacity

            a. The Wingate Anaerobic Test

            b. The Margaria-Kalamen Stair Climb

            c. Field Tests

III. The Anaerobic Exercise Response

    A. Oxygen Deficit and Excess Postexercise Oxygen Consumption

    B. ATP-PC Changes

    C. Lactate Changes

        1. The Lactate Threshold(s)

        2. Why Is Lactic Acid a Problem?

            a. Pain

            b. Performance Decrement

        3. The Fate of Lactate

        4. Lactate Removal Postexercise

IV. Male vs. Female Anaerobic Characteristics

    A. The Availability and Utilization of ATP-PC

    B. The Accumulation of Lactate

    C. Mechanical Power and Capacity

V. Anaerobic Exercise Characteristics of Children
   A. The Availability and Utilization of ATP-PC
   B. The Accumulation of Lactate
      1. The Muscle Enzyme Theory
      2. Sexual Maturation Theory
      3. Neurohormonal Regulation Theory
   C. The Lactate Threshold(s)
   D. Mechanical Power and Capacity
VI. Anaerobic Exercise Characteristics of Older Adults
   A. The Availability and Utilization of ATP-PC
   B. The Accumulation of Lactate
   C. Mechanical Power and Capacity
VII. Heritability of Anaerobic Characteristics

Chapter 10

CARDIOVASCULAR RESPONSE TO EXERCISE

Suggested Laboratory Activities

1. Time each student as she/he performs three of the following runs (comparable distance can of course be used if other modalities are selected):
   - 100 m dash
   - 200 m dash
   - 400 m dash
   - 800 m dash
   - 1500 or 1600 m run
   - 3 mile run

   On the basis of the performance times, determine the approximate percent contribution of aerobic and anaerobic metabolism using Figure 10.2.

2. Compare and contrast lactate accumulation ([La$^-$]) from the following activities:
   - 10 second Wingate Anaerobic Test (arms or legs)
   - 30 second Wingate Anaerobic Test (arms of legs)
   - 20 minute cycle ergometer ride (heart rate not to exceed 120 b·min^{-1})

3. Calculate the peak power, mean power, and Fatigue Index for contrasting individuals such as:
   - untrained male versus untrained female
   - aerobically trained versus anaerobically trained (same sex)
   - anaerobically trained athlete versus untrained individual (same sex)

4. Complete a single load submaximal aerobic workout. Measure oxygen consumption at rest (5 minutes), during exercise (20 minutes), and during recovery (15 minutes). Graph the results showing oxygen deficit and EPOC (Figure 10.5, p. 252).

5. Determine [La$^-$] every 5 minutes for 30 minutes during recovery from an interval training session. Use three recovery variations:
   - rest
   - walking
   - jogging at a self-selected pace

   Compare and contrast the results.

Chapter 10

ANAEROBIC METABOLISM DURING EXERCISE
Review Questions

1. Describe the energy continuum. For each of the following sports or events, determine the percentage contribution from the ATP-PC, LA, and O_2 systems.

    Figure 10.2; Pgs. 244-246
    The energy continuum indicates the relative contribution of each energy system (alactic anaerobic or ATP-PC; lactic anaerobic or LA; and aerobic or O_2) to the total energy requirements of an activity based on the time of the activity. This assumes that the intensity of all-out effort decreases from 100% to 80% as the duration of the activity increases from 10 seconds to 120 minutes.

Event	% ATP-PC	%LA	%O_2
100-m dash	75	10	15
800-m dash	30	50	20
soccer	20	20	60
triathlon	<1	<1	98
volleyball spike	100	0	0
100-m swim	17	58	25
mile run	2	8	80
stealing a base	65	10	15

2. List the major variables that are typically measured to describe the anaerobic response to exercise. Where possible, provide an example of an exercise test from which the variable could be determined.

Figure 10.7, 10.9; Table 10.2; Pgs. 246-258

Major Anaerobic Variables	Exercise Test Example
Chemical	
• ATP-PPC	• must be measured directly after high intensity exercise
• lactate concentration	• must be measured directly after high intensity exercise
• lactate thresholds (LT1 & LT2)	• Incremental test to maximum (cycle ergometer)
Mechanical work/ performance	
• mean power	• Wingate Anaerobic Test (WAT)
• peak power	• WAT/ Margaria-Kalamem Stair Climb/ vertical jump
• fatigue index	• WAT
• lactic anaerobic power & capacity	• sprint and middle distance run times
• alactic anaerobic power	• short (40-100-m) dash times

3. Explain the five physiological reasons for the production of lactic acid. What determines whether or not lactate accumulates in the blood?

   Pgs. 247-248, 270
   The five physiological reasons for the production of lactate are:
   a) anaerobiosis or lack of oxygen;
   b) the activity of lactate dehydrogenase is higher then that of the enzymes that provide alternate pathways for pyruvate;
   c) hormonal changes during exercise increase the breakdown of glycogen leading to increased G6P levels. In turn, glycolysis and the production of pyruvate are increased. High levels of pyruvate lead to high levels of lactate as noted in b;
   d) muscle contraction stimulates glycogenolysis and the sequence of events described in c;
   e) the recruitment of fast twitch muscle fibers, especially FG fibers.

4. Arrange the ATP-PC, LA, and O2 systems from highest to lowest in terms of (a) power and (b) capacity. What is the difference between power and capacity?

Table 10.1; Pgs. 248-249

	Power	Capacity
high	ATP-PC	O_2
medium	LA	LA
low	O_2	ATP-PC

In terms of the energy system, power is defined as the maximum amount of energy that can be produced per unit of time, and is expressed in kcal·min^{-1} (kJ·min^{-1}). Capacity is defined as the total amount of energy that can be produced by the energy system. It is expressed in kcal (kJ)

5. Diagram the oxygen deficit and excess postexercise oxygen consumption for an activity that requires 110% VO$_2$max in an individual whose VO$_2$ max equals 4 L·min^{-1}. Explain how energy is provided during the oxygen deficit time period and why oxygen remains elevated during recovery.

Figure 10.5; Pgs. 252-254

Energy is provided during the oxygen deficit by four sources: (1) O$_2$ transport and utilization; (2) utilization of oxygen stores in capillary blood and on myoglobin; (3) splitting of stored ATP-PC; (4) anaerobic glycolysis with the concomitant production of lactic acid. Energy remains elevated during the excess post exercise oxygen consumption (EPOC) phase because: (1) restoration of ATP-PC stores which have a half-life of 30 sec, so full storage takes about 2 min; (2) restoration of O$_2$ stores which takes about 2-3 min; (3) elevated cardiovascular-respiratory function accounts for 1-2% of excess O$_2$; (4) elevated hormonal levels (catecholamines, thyroxine, and cortisol); (5) elevated body temperature, which is the major factor; and (6) lactate removal.

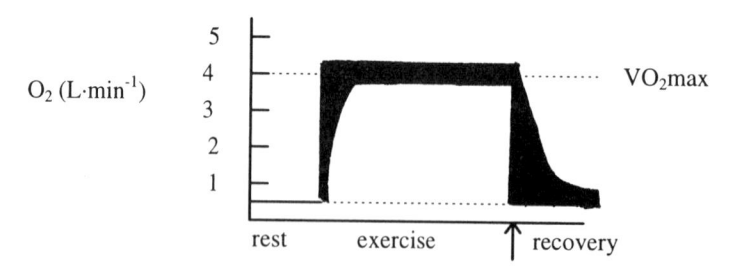

6. Diagram and explain the changes that take place in ATP, PC, and [LA⁻] during constant-load, heavy exercise lasting 3 minutes or less.

Figure 10.7; Table 10.3; Pg. 254
ATP, PC and Lactate changes in heavy exercise in <3 minutes are as follows: ATP level in the muscle decreases only slightly (30-40%). The greatest depletion of PC occurs in the first 20 seconds of exercise, after which the decline in both ATP and PC is gradual. PC is nearly depleted (decreased by 60-70%). Lactate level depends on intensity of exercise but in short duration high intensity exercise, lactate levels rise immediately at onset and continue throughout exercise, reading levels from 2-12 $mmol \cdot L^{-1}$.

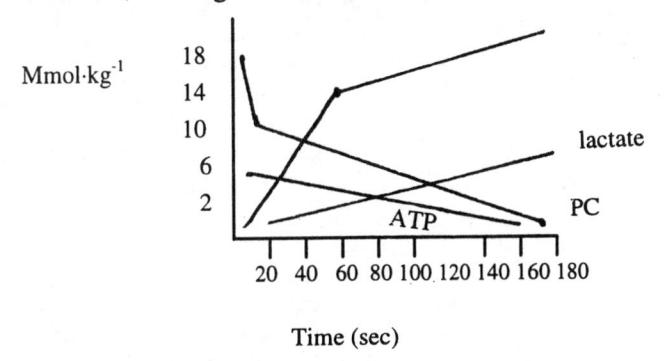

7. Diagram the lactate response to incremental work to maximum. The ventilatory and lactate thresholds often occur at approximately the same time. Debate whether this is a result of cause and effect or coincidence. Can either the lactate thresholds or the ventilatory thresholds be accurately described as anaerobic thresholds? Why or why not?

Figures 10.8, 10.9; Pgs. 248-255, 270

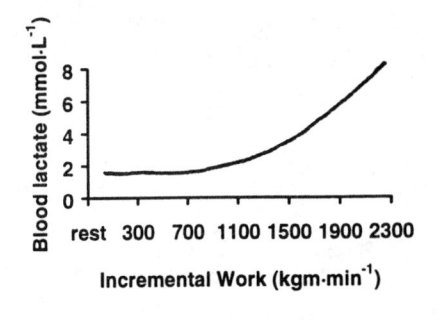

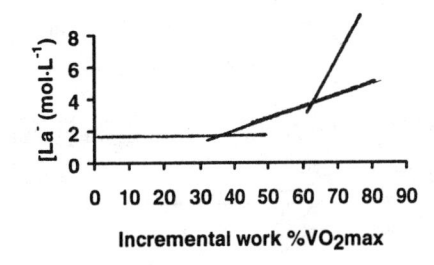

In order for the accumulation of lactate (indicated by the lactate thresholds) to be causally related to the breakpoints seen in minute ventilation (ventilatory thresholds) the following conditions must be met:

Condition	Evidence
Lactic acid or some by-product of it's buffering must be capable of stimulating respiration almost simultaneous to it's production	• **Pro**- Carbon dioxide is produced as a result of the buffering of lactic acid ($NaHCO_3$ + HLa $\leftrightarrow$ NaLa + H_2O; H_2CO_3 $\leftrightarrow$ H_2O + CO_2) CO_2 is a potent stimulant of respiration • **Con**- The presence of lactic acid is not the only mechanism that can account for an increase in CO_2 or V_E. For example, McArdle's syndrome patients cannot produce lactic acid due to an enzyme deficiency yet they show VT points.
Anything which affects the lactate threshold should affect the ventilatory thresholds equally	• **Con**- The LT and VT points do not change to the same extent in the same individuals as a result of training, glycogen depletion, and varying pedaling rates.

Neither the lactate thresholds nor the ventilatory thresholds can be accurately described as anaerobic thresholds.

- the presence of lactate does not automatically mean that there is a lack of oxygen (anaerobiosis). Instead, the presence of lactate instead reflects the use of the anaerobic glycolytic pathway (by fast twitch fibers and from the utilization of glycogen) and the balance between glycolytic and mitochondrial activity (the balance between lactate production, removal and clearance, as well as the rate of pyruvate oxidation). Most importantly, lactate accumulation does not occur at the time of increased production.
- the pattern of lactate accumulation is more likely a positive exponential curve than any sharp breakpoints or thresholds.

8. What are the physiological effects of lactate accumulation?

Pgs. 258-260
The physiological effects of lactic acid are more related to the concentration of H^+ ions than the concentration of La^-. The effects of an increased concentration of H^+ on the decrease in pH include: pain, performance decrement, reduced production of ATP (rate-limiting enzymes can be inactivated, and substrate availability is inhibited); reduced force and velocity of muscle contraction by:

[1] inhibition of actomyosin ATPase which is the enzyme responsible for the breakdown of ATP for muscle contraction, and
[2] interference with the actions and uptake of calcium ions that is necessary for excitation-coupling and relaxation of protein cross-bridges within muscle fibers. High levels of lactate ions may also interfere with cross bridging.

9. What happens to lactic acid during exercise and recovery? What is the best way to clear lactate quickly during recovery?

Table 10.4; pg. 260
Lactic acid/lactate has two major fates during exercise and recovery:
- it serves as a fuel source for both cardiac and slow twitch muscle fibers, either by diffusing directly into adjacent muscle fibers or into the venous circulation and traveling to these cells. Prior to use, it is converted to pyruvate. The process accounts for approximately 55-70% of the lactate removal.
- the carbon structure of lactate is converted to other structures through gluconeogenic or transamination processes, forming glucose, glycogen and keto acids (20%) or amino acids (5-10%). Less than 2% remains as lactate.

Active recovery is the best way to clear lactate quickly during recovery. Continuous activity is best at intensity levels below the lactate threshold (~29-45% VO_2max for cycling and 55-70% VO_2max for running).

10. What are the effects of sex and age on anaerobic metabolism during exercise?

Figures 10.14, 10.16, 10.18; Pgs. 262-269

The Influence of Age on Anaerobic Metabolism

Variable	Children	Young Adults	Elderly
ATP-PC	• no difference per kg of muscle mass but less muscle mass total • no difference in utilization during exercise	baseline for comparison	stores are reduced an unable to be used quickly
[La⁻]max	lower	baseline for comparison	lower
LT2	lower absolute workload but higher %VO_2max	baseline for comparison	unknown
Mechanical Power & Capacity	lower	baseline for comparison	lower

The Influence of Sex on Anaerobic Metabolism

Variable	Female	Male
ATP-PC	• no difference per kg of muscle mass but males have greater muscle mass • no difference in utilization during exercise	baseline for comparison
[La⁻]max	lower	baseline for comparison
LT1 & LT2	same %VO2max lower absolute workload	baseline for comparison
Mechanical Power & Capacity	• lower peak power & mean power • equal fatigue index	baseline for comparison

11. Approximately how much of an individual's anaerobic ability is due to genetics? Are sprinters made or born?

   Pg. 269
   Approximately 44-76% of an individual's anaerobic ability is due to genetics, the exact amount is unknown. At least to a certain extent, sprinters are born.

Chapter 10

ANAEROBIC METABOLISM DURING EXERCISE
Exam Questions

A. Multiple Choice

1. Which of the following statements is valid?
   a. At the breaking of the tape, a 4 min miler has depleted his CP but not ATP phosphagen resources, attained a maximum oxygen consumption, and incurred a degree of lactic acid build-up at the extremes of tolerance.
   b. At the braking of the tape, a 4 min. miler has reserves of phosphagen resources (ATP, CP), attained a maximum oxygen consumption, and has resynthesized any lactic acid that might have been created during the race.
   c. At the breaking of the tape, a 4 min. miler has depleted his phosphagen resources (ATP, CP), is working submaximally in terms of oxygen consumption, and has incurred a degree of lactic acid build-up at the extremes of tolerance.
   d. At the breaking of the tape, a 4 min. miler has depleted his phosphagen resources (ATP, CP), attained a maximum oxygen consumption, and has resynthesized any lactic acid that might have been created during the race.

Answer- a

2. O_2 deficit:
   a. is the amount of oxygen taken up in recovery in excess of resting use, the EPOC.
   b. is usually larger after endurance training than before due to the higher work capacity after training.
   c. depends for energy on the splitting of ATP/PC, oxygen bound to myoglobin and anaerobic glycolysis.
   d. results from increased body temperature and hormonal levels.

Answer- c

3. An analysis of the energy continuum indicates that:
   a. ATP-PC, LA and O_2 system are all involved in providing energy for all durations of exercise.
   b. The ATP-PC portion of anaerobic metabolism predominates in activities lasting 10 sec or less, while the LA portion of anaerobic metabolism is most important between 10-30 sec and 2-3 minutes of activity.
   c. By 5 minutes of exercise, the O_2 system is clearly dominant and the longer the duration the more important it becomes.
   d. a, b, and c are correct.

Answer- d

4. The accepted explanation for the O_2 deficit is that :
   a. the respiratory system is unable to respond quickly enough to the increased need for O_2.
   b. the cardiovascular system is unable to respond quickly enough to the increased energy demands.
   c. the by-products of the additional energy use (ADP, P_i and NADH + H^+) stimulate both aerobic and anaerobic metabolism.
   d. the muscle mitochondria are unable to respond quickly enough to the increased energy demands.

Answer- c

5. The most important physiological reason for EPOC is:
   a. elevated body temperature.
   b. restoration of myoglobin O_2 stores and ATP-PC stores.
   c. elevated cardiorespiratory and hormonal levels.
   d. lactate removal.

Answer- a

6. Which of the following recovery patterns should be recommended for a middle distance runner at a conference meet? On day 1 she must do a preliminary heat in both the 400 m and 800 m run. One hour separates these heats.
   a. Rest between the heats; eat a high carbohydrate energy bar and ingest a sports drink.
   b. Jog for about 20 min at a moderate intensity after the first heat, then rest and consume a fluid of choice.
   c. Walk slowly for most of the time between heats while ingesting water.
   d. Stretch and do light calisthenics between heats, ingest fluid about 10 min before the second heat.

Answer- b

7. A lactate level of approximately 10 mmol · L⁻¹ would indicate:
   a. a normal resting lactate level for a well trained male or female athlete.
   b. the results of a maximal workload.
   c. the results of a submaximal workload.
   d. insufficient oxygen to create enough ATP to carry out the workload.

Answer- b

8. As a fitness leader you are asked to test the anaerobic power of the football team. You decide to use the following test:
   a. 12 minute run test, with a sprint a the end
   b. 1 repetition max in the squat
   c. 1 mile run
   d. Wingate

Answer- d

9. Lactate serves the following functions during recovery from exercise:
   a. It keeps the subject from exercising too soon before an adequate recovery has been achieved.
   b. It serves as a carbon source for other substances.
   c. It serves as a fuel source.
   d. b and c
   e. none of the above are correct.

Answer- d

B. Fill in the Blank

1. _____ _____ _____ is the total amount of energy that can be produced by an energy system.
   Answer- Energy System Capacity

2. _____ _____ _____ is the maximal amount of energy that can be produced per unit of time.
   Answer- Energy System Power

3. _____ _____ is defined as the maximum power (force times distance divided by time) exerted during very short (5 sec or less) duration work.
   Answer- Peak Power

4. The average power (force times distance divided by time) exerted during short- (typically 30 sec) duration work is _____ _____.
   Answer- Mean Power

5. The Percentage of peak power drop-off during high-intensity, short-duration work is called _____ _____.
Answer- Fatigue Index

6. _____ _____ is the difference between the oxygen required during exercise and the oxygen supplied and utilized. Occurs at the onset of all activity.
Answer- Oxygen Deficit

7. Oxygen consumption during recovery that is above normal resting values is called _____ _____ _____ _____.
Answer- Excess Postexercise Oxygen consumption

8. The _____ _____ are points on the linear-curvilinear continuum of lactate accumulation that appear to indicate sharp rises, often labeled as the first (LT1) and second (LT2) lactate threshold.
Answer- Lactate Thresholds

Chapter 11

AEROBIC METABOLISM DURING EXERCISE

Outline

I. Introduction

II. Laboratory Measurement of Aerobic Metabolism

   A. Calorimetry

   B. Spirometry

III. Aerobic Exercise Responses

   A. Oxygen Consumption and Carbon Dioxide Production

      1. Short-Term, Light-to Moderate-Intensity Submaximal Exercise

      2. Prolonged, Moderate to Heavy Submaximal Exercise

      3. Incremental Exercise to Maximum

      4. Static and Dynamic-Resistance Exercise

   B. The Oxygen Cost of Breathing

   C. Respiratory Quotient/Respiratory Exchange Ratio

   D. Lactate Changes

   E. Estimation of Caloric Intake and Expenditure

   F. The Metabolic Equivalent (MET)

IV. Field Estimates of Energy Expenditure During Exercise

   A. Metabolic Calculations Based on Mechanical Work or Standard Energy Use

   B. Motion Sensors and Accelerometers

   C. Activity Recalls and Questionnaires

V. Efficiency and Economy

   A. Efficiency

   B. Economy of Walking and Running

      1. The Influence of Sex on Economy

    2. The Influence of Age on Economy
VI. Why Do Economy and Efficiency Matter?
VII. Heritability of Aerobic Characteristics

… Chapter 11

AEROBIC METABOLISM DURING EXERCISE
Suggested Laboratory Activities

1. Measure oxygen consumption while performing the following exercises and during 5 minutes of recovery:
    - walk on the treadmill at 3.5 mi·hr^{-1} at 0% grade for 10 minutes
    - run on the treadmill at 6 mi·hr^{-1} at 3% grade for 45 minutes
    - an incremental test to maximum on the treadmill
    - static handgrip with maximal effort for 2 minutes
    - 1 set of 8 reps at 75% 1-RM of 2 arm biceps curls

Graph, describe, and discuss the results.

2. Compute the RER for selected minutes of the above exercise sessions or any other exercise session of choice, and relate these values to fuel utilization.

3. Determine the caloric cost of at least 2 of the exercise sessions from number 1 or any other activity of choice.

4. Compare and contrast lactate accumulation using one recovery sample from each exercise session in number 1.

5. Verify, using physiological criteria, whether an incremental test was truly maximal or not.

6. Determine the MET level for the exercise session in number 1 or any activity of choice.

7. Determine the gross, net, and delta efficiency on the treadmill, cycle ergometer, Stair Master, Nordic Track or some other selected modality.

8. Determine and compare/contrast the velocity at VO$_2$max of two individuals in the class. Discuss the practical application of the results in terms of a 10 km run competition between the two.

Chapter 11

AEROBIC METABOLISM DURING EXERCISE
Review Questions

1. List the variables used to describe the aerobic metabolic response to exercise. Describe how each one is obtained from laboratory or field tests. Explain what each variable means.

   Table 11.1, 11.2, 11.5; Pgs. 276-287, 289-292

Variable	Meaning	Obtained
oxygen consumed (VO_2 cons)	amount of oxygen taken up, transported and used in cellular respiration	open-circuit indirect spirometry, standardized formula based on mechanical work
carbon dioxide produced (VCO_2 prod)	amount of carbon dioxide produced as by product of cellular respiration	open-circuit indirect spirometry
respiratory exchange (RER)	ratio of VCO_2/VO_2 which indicates relative carbohydrate and fat substrate utilization	open-circuit indirect spirometry
caloric cost (kcal or kcal·min^{-1})	amount of energy expended that is dependent on aerobic metabolism	open-circuit indirect spirometry, charts
MET level	multiples of resting seated energy expenditure	open-circuit indirect spirometry, charts

2. Diagram the oxygen consumption response during (a) short term, light-to-moderate intensity, dynamic exercise; (b) prolonged, moderate to heavy submaximal exercise; and (c) incremental exercise to maximum.

   Figure 11.4; Pgs. 280-282

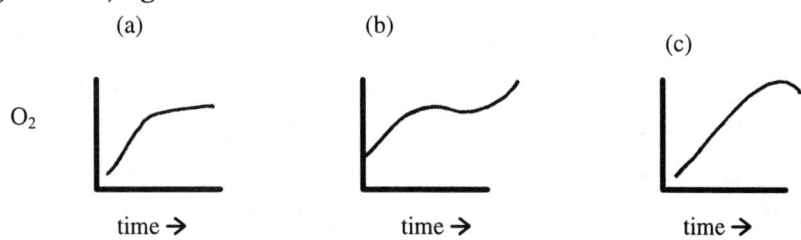

3. Describe the relationship between the oxygen cost of breathing and exercise intensity.

   Pgs. 283-284
   The oxygen cost of breathing and the intensity of exercise go hand in hand. Some oxygen that is used is for the respiratory muscles. At rest, the respiratory system uses about 1-2 % of oxygen consumption(2.5 mL·min^{-1}). During light exercise where the V_E is less than 60 L·min^{-1}, the oxygen cost changes minimally (25 - 100 mL·min^{-1}). During heavy exercise where V_E is between 60 - 120 L·min^{-1} then the oxygen response may rise from 50 to 400 mL·min^{-1}. During incremental exercise to maximum the initial oxygen cost of breathing shows a very gradual curvilinear rise, reflecting the submaximal changes note previously. At workloads above those requiring a V_E greater than 120 L·min^{-1} a dramatic exponential curve occurs in the oxygen cost of breathing rising from 3 to 13% of the VO_2 used in exercise.

4. Explain the respiratory quotient and the respiratory exchange ratio. Relate them to the determination of energy substrate utilization, theoretically and numerically.

   Tables 11.3, 11.4; Pgs. 284-287
   Both the respiratory quotient (RQ) and the respiratory exchange ratio (RER) are computed from the formula VCO_2/VO_2. The RQ reflects what is occurring on the cellular utilization level and can be obtained for carbohydrate, fat and protein using mole or molecules. The RER is obtained from total body open circuit indirect spirometry measures. The RER indicates the relative percentage of calories expended from carbohydrate and fat but not protein. The RQ represents just fuel utilization; the RER represents fuel utilization confounded by anaerobic metabolism, non-working muscle metabolism and non-metabolic CO_2. The metabolic range of both is from 0.7 to 1.0.

	RQ	**RER**
Carbohydrate	1.0	0.85= 49%; 1.0= 100%
Fat	0.7	0.7= 100%; 0.85= 51%
Protein	0.74 (BCAA) - 0.81 (PRO)	cannot determine

5. Compare lactate accumulation during (a) dynamic, short term, light-to-moderate - intensity exercise and (b) prolonged, moderate to heavy exercise. Contrast these responses to the short-term, high-intensity dynamic anaerobic exercise and incremental exercise to maximum detailed in the previous chapter.

   Figures 11.6, 11.7, 11.8, 11.8; Table 11.5; Pgs. 287-289

Exercise Task	Lactate Accumulation
dynamic, short term, light-to-moderate intensity	slight initial increase during the oxygen deficit period; barely exceeds resting values
prolonged, moderate to heavy exercise	after an initial rise, during the oxygen deficit period the [La$^-$] may stay the same or decrease slightly remaining close to resting values
short-term, high intensity dynamic anaerobic exercise	large increase in [La$^-$] with values much greater than resting (8-12 mmol·L^{-1} range)
incremental exercise to maximum	positive exponential curvilinear rise or rectilinear rise with two break points to values exceeding 8 mmol·L^{-1}

6. Explain the similarities and differences in describing activity by kilocalories and MET levels. How can both be practically applied?

   Table 11.6, 11.7; Pgs. 289-292
   Describing physical activity by kcal and MET levels is similar because both are based on oxygen consumption and both express energy expenditure. METs are based on an approximate resting values of 3.5ml kg min and all activity is then expressed as a multiple of a resting MET value of 1. Caloric cost requires some knowledge of an RER values. Exercise prescription can be based on either using available charts. Estimate of energy expenditure are important for weight control, etc.

7. Differentiate, in terms of definition, calculation, and application, between gross efficiency, net efficiency and delta efficiency. How can a cyclist maximize his or her efficiency?

Pgs. 294-299

Variable	Definition	Calculation % (x 100)	Application
Gross Efficiency	The percentage of energy input that appears as useful external work	$\dfrac{\text{work output}}{\text{energy expend}}$	Used when calculating values for specific workloads, in nutritional studies
Net Efficiency	The energy expended is corrected for resting metabolic rate	$\dfrac{\text{work output}}{\text{energy expend - RMR}}$	When only the efficiency of the work bout itself is wanted
Delta Efficiency	Is the efficiency based on the difference between two workloads	$\dfrac{\text{difference in work output between 2 loads}}{\text{difference in energy expenditure between the same 2 loads}}$	When a relative indication of energy cost from an additional work load is wanted

A cyclist can maximize their efficiency by adjusting seat height to 109% of leg length, pedal frequency to between 40 and 60 rev·min^{-1}, and drafting off of other cyclists.

8. Compare running economy by sex and age. Discuss possible reasons for any observed differences. Give three situations where any observed differences could have significant practical meaning.

Figures 11.12, 11.13; Pgs. 298-304
The influence of sex on the interindividual variation in economy is unclear. However, even if the oxygen cost is equal at any given speed, the female typically has a lower VO$_2$max and hence will be working at a higher % VO$_2$max at any given speed. Practical significance- the female is likely to be unable to run at as fast a pace in a long distance event as a male. Children and adolescents are less economical than adults; the elderly may be less economical than young and middle-aged adults.

Possible reasons for the lower economy in children include:
- Children have a higher basal/resting metabolic rate than adults, hence gross exercise oxygen consumption may be higher because RMR is higher.
- Children have a greater surface area per unit of mass than adults which necessitates a higher RMR to maintain body temperature.
- Children exhibit immature running mechanics, however, the only one likely to impact oxygen cost is the higher stride frequency. When one stride is considered, the oxygen cost does not differ between children and adults. However, at any given pace the child has a higher number of strides, thus using more energy both to accelerate and brake the body's mass.
- Children have a higher ventilatory equivalent than adults. The processing of this additional air requires additional energy.
- Children are less able to generate ATP anaerobically than adults. Adults may provide more energy anaerobically (even at submaximal exercise levels) than children do.

Practical significance:
- children are at a disadvantage (e.g. must work at a higher %VO_2max) when running with or competing against more mature children, adolescents or adults.
- performance on tests of cardiovascular fitness will improve as children mature despite no change in VO_2max.
- adult prediction equations based on VO_2/speed relationships to predict VO_2max cannot be used for children.

9. Show how efficiency or economy can have an impact on exercise performance.

Higher efficiency, such as in cycling, should increase performance; higher economy is running should do the same, if the event is endurance in nature. If two runners have the same VO_2max and can run at the same percentage of the VO_2max, the more economical runner will have a definite advantage. The velocity at VO_2max or the speed at which an individual can run when working at his or her VO_2max which is based on both economy and VO_2max may be the most important predictor of endurance performance.

10. Describe the impact of genetics on aerobic metabolism.
    There appears to be a significant genetic effect at low work intensities, not at high intensities.

Workload (watts, W)	Genetic Influence (%)
50	90
75	78
100	46
125	not significant
150	not significant

Chapter 11

AEROBIC METABOLISM DURING EXERCISE
Exam Questions

A. Multiple Choice

1. An individual uses 1.2 l/min of O_2 and produces 1.12 l/min of CO_2. His/her RER is:
   a. 1.07
   b. .75
   c. .93
   d. .82

   Answer- c

2. The individual whose RER you just calculated is:
   a. in an anaerobic state.
   b. burning primarily carbohydrate as a fuel.
   c. burning a mixed diet.
   d. burning primarily fat as a fuel.

   Answer- b

3. When an individual exercises or otherwise performs external work:
   a. the actual work represents only a portion of the total energy utilized.
   b. the energy not used to perform the work appears as heat and must be dissipated or the body temperature will rise.
   c. the percentage of energy input which appears as useful external work is called the economy of the task.
   d. a and b are correct.

   Answer-d

4. Which of the following statements represents the best advice and physiological reasoning for a cyclist racing into a headwind?
   a. Slowly work your way to the head of the pack so as not to accumulate large quantities of lactate early, but then hold the lead.
   b. Tuck in behind another cyclist going about your race pace to minimize the energy needed to overcome the air resistance, then sprint to the finish ahead of that (and other) cyclists
   c. Aim for a negative split (a faster second half than a first half) to avoid carrying an oxygen deficit whether you ride alone or beside another rider.
   d. Make your bike and yourself as aerodynamically smooth as possible (helmet, position, wheels, etc.), and just go for it!

Answer- b

5. Use the following information to determine the caloric expenditure if this individual exercises at the indicated level for 30 minutes.

   $\dot{V}O_2 = 1.85$ L·min^{-1} Caloric equivalent = 4.948 kcal·LO$_2$$^{-1}$

   $\dot{V}O_2 = 33$ ml·kg^{-1}·min   RER = 0.92

   a. 163 kcal
   b. 275 kcal
   c. 304 kcal
   d. 915 kcal

Answer- b

6. What is the MET level of the exercise described in the last question?
   a. 3.5
   b. 5.6
   c. 7.8
   d. 9.4

Answer- d

7. Given the following information, determine if this test was a maximal effort.
   Gender: female   age: 40 yr.   HR max: 178 b·min^{-1} RPE: 20
   length of test: 12 min.   lactate: 9.2 mmol·L^{-1} change in O$_2$ consumption from minute 11 to minute 12: increased 1.5 ml·kg^{-1}·min^{-1}
   a. it was a maximal effort
   b. cannot tell from the information provided
   c. it was a peak effort, cannot call it a maximal effort
   d. cannot tell, must observe the test in person to see the subject's effort

Answer- a

8. Gross efficiency is:
   a. [energy expended X work output] X 100.
   b. [work output / energy input] X 100.
   c. [work output / energy expended] X 100.
   d. someone who gets all of their work done before it is due.

Answer- c

9. As children become older there is a decline in the O_2 consumption of relative work and therefore, a progressive increase in economy of work. Which of the following may help explain this phenomena?
   a. the Surface Law
   b. the older we become, the more practice we have in walking
   c. an increase in BMR occurs as we get older
   d. none of these offer any explanation to the phenomena

Answer- a

10. The difference between RQ and RER is
    a. one represents the ratio of CO_2 and O_2 at the cellular level, while the other represents the ration of CO_2 and O_2 in expired air.
    b. no difference exists. They are 2 different names for the same thing.
    c. approximately 10%.
    d. one represents the difference that exists when a subject is not in a fasted condition prior to the onset of an exercise test.

Answer- a

11. Which of the following statements is not true regarding metabolism when comparing children to adults?
    a. At any given submaximal pace, children will be working at a higher percent of their $\dot{V}O_{2max}$ than the adult.
    b. Children have a lower glycolytic capacity than do adults possibly due to lower levels of phosphofructokinase.
    c. In children, endurance performance parallels running economy whereas in adults, endurance performance is more dependent on $\dot{V}O_{2max}$.
    d. At any given submaximal pace, children & adults exhibit the same running economy.

Answer- d

B. Fill in the Blank

1. The measurement of heat energy liberated or absorbed in metabolic processes is _____.
   Answer- Calorimetry

2. _____ is an indirect calorimetry method for estimating heat production or calorimetry in which expired air is measured and analyzed for the amount of oxygen consumed and carbon dioxide produced.
   Answer- Spirometry

3. The amount of oxygen taken up, transported, and used at the cellular level is called _____ _____.
   Answer- Oxygen Consumption

4. _____ is the term that describes the amount of carbon dioxide generated during metabolism.
   Answer- Carbon Dioxide Produced

5. The term _____ _____ describes a situation that occurs in submaximal activity of long duration, or above 70% VO$_2$max, or in hot and humid conditions where the oxygen consumption increases, despite the fact that the oxygen requirement of the activity has not changed.
   Answer- Oxygen Drift

6. The highest amount of oxygen an individual can take in and utilize to produce ATP aerobically while breathing air during heavy exercise is called _____ _____ _____.
   Answer- Maximal Oxygen Consumption

7. The _____ _____ is the ratio of the amount of carbon dioxide produced divided by the amount of oxygen consumed at the cellular level.
   Answer- Respiratory Quotient

8. The ratio of the volume of CO_2 produced divided by the volume of O_2 consumed is called the _____ _____ _____.
   Answer- Respiratory Exchange Ratio

9. _____ _____ is the number of kilocalories produced per liter of oxygen consumed.
   Answer- Caloric Equivalent

10. Energy expenditure of an activity performed for a specified period of time is called _____ _____.
    Answer- Caloric Cost

11. A _____ is a unit that represents the metabolic equivalent of multiples in the resting rate of oxygen consumption of any given activity.
    Answer- MET

12. The percentage of energy input that appears as useful external work is called _____ _____.
    Answer- Mechanical Efficiency

13. _____ is the oxygen cost of walking or running at varying speeds.
    Answer- Economy

14. The speed at which an individual can run when working at his or her maximal oxygen consumption is called _____.
    Answer- Velocity at VO$_2$max

Chapter 12

Metabolic Training Principles and Adaptations

Outline

I. Introduction

II. Application of the Training Principles for Metabolic Enhancement

    A. Specificity

    B. Overload

        1. The Time or Distance Technique

            a. ATP-PC System

            b. LA System

            c. O_2 System

        2. The Lactate Monitoring Technique

    C. Adaptation

    D. Progression

    E. Individualization

    F. Maintenance

    G. Retrogression/Plateau/Reversibility

    H. Warm-Up and Cool-Down

III. Metabolic Adaptations to Exercise Training

    A. Substrate or Fuel Supply

        1. Regulatory Hormones

        2. Carbohydrate

        3. Fat

        4. Protein

    B. Enzyme Activity

        1. Glycolytic Enzymes

          a. Hexokinase

          b. Phosphorylase

          c. Phosphofructokinase (PFK)

          d. Lactic Dehydrogenase (LDH)

      2. Shuttles

      3. Mitochondrial Enzymes

  C. Oxygen Utilization

      1. Maximal Oxygen Uptake

      2. Submaximal Oxygen Cost

      3. Oxygen Deficit and Drift

  D. Lactate Accumulation

  E. ATP Production, Storage, and Turnover

      1. ATP-PC

      2. Work Output

IV. The Influence of Age and Sex on Metabolic Training Adaptations

V. The Impact of Genetics on Metabolic Trainability

  A. Submaximal Substrate or Fuel Utilization

  B. Maximal Work Output and Oxygen Consumption

  C. Genetic Variability

Chapter 12

METABOLIC TRAINING PRINCIPLES AND ADAPTATIONS
Suggested Laboratory Activities

1. Have students write a metabolic training program that incorporates both anaerobic and aerobic components and explain how each training principle is used in it.

2. Have students write a periodization cycle showing variations in metabolic intensity, frequency, and duration for an aerobic sport and an anaerobic sport.

3. Have students exercise (using a modality of choice) for 5 continuous minutes at each of the following steady state heart rates:
   - 100-110 b·min^{-1}
   - 120 b·min^{-1}
   - 160 b·min^{-1}
   - 5 minutes of exercise time of interval work at 170-180 b·min^{-1}

After each 5 minute bout measure lactate accumulation. Have each individual determine if she/he can monitor the metabolic intensity or work-outs by using the guidelines established on p. 312.

4. Have students perform the Conconi test using an exercise modality of choice. Measure [La$^-$] at the point of heart rate deflection. Have each student determine if the heart rate at this deflection represents 4 mmol·L^{-1}. Some students may not show a deflection. Have them discuss possible reasons for this and what it means from a practical standpoint.

5. Compare and contrast oxygen consumption, oxygen deficit, RER, substrate utilization, oxygen drift, excess post exercise oxygen consumption and lactate accumulation during an absolute submaximal exercise session among an aerobically trained, a dynamic resistance trained, and an untrained individual of the same sex.

Chapter 12

METABOLIC TRAINING PRINCIPLES AND ADAPTATIONS
Review Questions

1. Name and briefly describe the eight training principles. Select a sport or fitness activity and show how each of the training principle can be specifically applied to that activity.

    Pgs. 310-315
    - *Specificity* begins with a determination of a goal. Once this is set, it is possible to determine the relative contributions of the energy systems. Generally, by stressing the primary systems during exercise, one can expect improvement. Specificity also applies to the major muscle groups and modality.
    - *Overload* is achieved in two ways: by manipulating time and distance, and by monitoring lactic acid levels. The time/distance technique involves continuos and/or interval training. The interval training relies on three major elements: a selected work interval (usually a distance), a target time and a predetermined recovery period. The energy system stressed is based on the length of the interval workout affecting the ATP-CP system (< 30 seconds), the LA system (30 seconds - 3 minutes), and the Oxygen system (> 3-5 minutes).
    - *Adaptation* is evident when a given distance or workload can be covered in a faster time with an equal or lower perception of fatigue or exertion and/or in the same time span with less physiological disruption and faster recovery. The key to adaptation for energy production in muscles appears to be allowing for sufficient recovery time between hard-intensity workouts.
    - *Progression* If further improvement is desired, then one can increase distance or workload, increase the number of repetitions or sessions, or decrease the length of the recovery interval or change the frequency of the various types of workouts per week. The key to progression is and increase in intensity and total training volume. It is also important for the progression to be gradual as a rule of thumb, no more than 10% increase per week.

- *Individualization* (1) Individualize according to the goal, (2) evaluate the individual, (3) develop periodization for the different seasons, (4) develop a format, that is the number of days per week devoted to each type of training or energy system stressed, and (5) determine training load based on the individual's evaluation and modified by how he/she responds and adapts.
- *Maintenance* is simply keeping oneself at a selected fitness level. One may even decrease the time and duration of the exercise as long as intensity is maintained. However, if there is a decrease in intensity, then there is a reduction in training adaptation. An athlete may taper prior to an important competition.
- *Retrogression/Plateau/Reversibility* At some point, an individual may fail to improve with progression and will either stay at the same level or decline. This may be a sign of overtraining. If the individual stops training all together, then detraining occurs. These metabolic factors that show the greatest improvement with training also show the greatest reversal with detraining.
- *Warm-up/Cool-down* The warm-up should elevate muscle temperature which will increase the rate at which the metabolic processes occur in the cells. The cool down phase allows lactic acid to dissipate faster during recovery and is maximized if the moderate intensity after exercise continues for 20 minutes.

Students may select any sport or position to show application of the training principles, hence their answers will differ widely. However, they should deal very specifically with each element of any given technique in each principle. For example, if monitoring by [La⁻] is chosen as the overload technique, activities that vary from < 2 mmol·L⁻¹ should be suggested.

2. Describe and explain the metabolic adaptations to exercise training for each of the following factors:
   (b) Substrate or fuel supply
   (c) Enzyme activity
   (d) Oxygen utilization
   (e) Lactate accumulation
   (f) ATP production, storage, and turnover

   Table 12.2; Pgs. 316-323
   (a) *Substrate or Fuel Supply* Regulatory hormones are a primary adaptation in the regulation of metabolism. During submaximal absolute or relative activity, hormonal response is blunted: the rise in glucagon is lower and the suppression of insulin is less;

the rise in norepinephrine, epinephrine, growth hormone, and cortisol is less. Muscle and liver glycogen reserves decrease. Trained individuals also use less CHO in his/her fuel mixture enabling him/her to sustain activity longer as glycogen is not as quickly depleted. (Sprinters, on the other hand, have an increased rate of glycogenolysis, giving these athletes a faster supply of substrate). Adaptation in fat metabolism occurs as: (a) an increased mobilization or release of free fatty acids from the adipose tissue, (b) an increased level of circulating plasma free fatty acids during submaximal exercise, (c) an increase in fat storage adjacent to the mitochondria within the muscles, and (d) an increased capacity to utilize fat at any given plasma concentration. The reliance as fat a fuel is called "glycogen sparing". There also exist an increased ability to utilize the branched chained amino acid leucine and the increased capacity to form alanine and release it from muscle cells.

(b) *Enzyme Activity* This is the key to increasing the production of ATP. (1) Glycolytic enzymes are involved in both the aerobic and anaerobic production of energy. Four enzymes that show adaptations include: (a) Hexokinase, which facilitates entry of glucose from the blood into the glycolytic pathway shows increased activity with endurance training; (b) Phosphorylase, which catalyses the breakdown of glycogen stored in muscle cells so glycogen may be used as fuel in glycolysis exhibits an increase with sprint training; (c) Phosphofructokinase, which is the main rate limiting enzyme of glycolysis shows an increase in activity with adequate levels of training; and (d) Lactic dehydrogenase which catalyses the conversion of pyruvate to lactic acid exhibits two adaptations; the overall activity of LDH is lowered and a shift occurs from the muscle to the heart form. (2) There are no training changes in the glycerol phosphate shuttle enzymes in skeletal muscle, but there is a large increase in enzymes in the malate-aspartate shuttle in the heart muscle. (3) Mitochodrial Enzymes of the Kreb cycle and the ETS are coupled with changes in the mitochondrial themselves. The size and number of the mitochondrial increase with training, and there is an overall greater enzyme activity. However, no cell mitochondrial enzymes increase to the same extent.

(c) *Oxygen utilization* (1) VO_2max increases with training. (2) Submax VO_2 remains the same for an absolute workload where no skill is involved where efficiency can change. (3) Oxygen deficit and drift. Oxygen deficit decreases in trained athletes due to oxidative phosphorylation being activated sooner. Oxygen drift is also less in a trained individual due to reductions in catecholamines, lactate accumulation and body temperature.

(d) *Lactate Accumulation.* Because less CHO is utilized during submaximal exercise in an athlete, less pyruvate is available for conversion into lactate. Higher workloads can be done before the 2 mmol·L^{-1} and 4 mmol·L^{-1} levels are reached. At maximal work the level of [La^{-1}] is higher after training due to greater glycogen supplies and increased activity of glycolytic enzymes, other than LDH. Both high [FFA] in cytoplasm and high levels of citrate cause the rate limiting enzyme PFK to slow down glycolysis and thus decreases the production of HLA. Lactate clearance is also higher in trained athletes due to an enhanced blood flow to the liver which aids in lactate removal.

(e) *ATP Production, Storage, and Turnover* The amount of ATP and CP stored in the resting muscle is higher in trained individuals, especially if muscle mass increases. There is also less depletion of them at the same absolute work loads but is unchanged in relative workloads. Therefore, the rate of turnover of ATP and CP increases.

3. Discuss the impact of genetics on the metabolic adaptations to exercise training in terms of the following factors:
   (c) submaximal substrate or fuel utilization
   (d) maximal work output and oxygen consumption
   (e) variability of response

Derive a practical application from this discussion, and provide a realistic example.

Pgs. 323-324
The impact of genetics on trainability is stronger than the heritability of the trait itself in sedentary individuals. The influence of genetics is also sometimes stronger the closer the individual is to achieving his/her maximal potential:
a) Adaptations in substrate availability and utilization as a result of endurance training are largely genetic, especially the ability to mobilize fat.
b) Long term, lactic, anaerobic and aerobic metabolic training adaptations are influenced more by genetics than are short-term. Alactic anaerobic adaptations (approximately 70-80% versus 30% of the variance accounted for).
c) Extreme variability (16-97% change) occurs in endurance performance as a result of the same training program. There may be as much as a 3-10 fold variation between high an low responders. Some people (~5% of the population) maybe non-responders. Some individuals respond quickly and others more slowly.

The application and example should involve the individualization principle and probably progression and overload.

Chapter 12

METABOLIC TRAINING PRINCIPLES AND ADAPTATIONS
Exam Questions

A. **Multiple Choice**

1. The most specific training for metabolic improvement should occur in which phase of the training cycle?
    a. pre-season
    b. during the season
    c. post season
    d. all year round

Answer-a

2. Overload of the metabolic system can be monitored by:
    a. RPE levels
    b. RQ levels
    c. Lactic acid levels
    d. HR levels

Answer- c

3. As a fitness expert, the local high school coach asks you to help train the 800 meter runners. Knowing that you need to train by overloading both the aerobic and anaerobic systems, you devise which of the following programs?
    a. super circuit weight training
    b. fartlek work out
    c. LSD work out
    d. 1 mile repeats

Answer- b

4. The same high school track coach asks you about the use of cross-training for her athletes. You reply:
    a. "Great training aid, but make sure your athletes always wear running shoes."
    b. "Great training aid for the cardiovascular system. It helps to reduce muskoskeletal stress, but is not as beneficial for the metabolic system."
    c. "Great training aid, but only if you can maintain heart rate max for longer than 10 minutes."
    d. "An overrated training aid that has been commercialized by professional athletes."

Answer- b

5. Taper training is a systematic reduction in training volume that allows for recovery from previous training, and helps "peak" athletes for competition. The taper should last:
    a. 1-2 days.
    b. 1-2 weeks.
    c. 1-2 months.
    d. only 1 day for each minute of competition.

Answer- e

6. A metabolic benefit of warming up prior to exercise is:
    a. a decreased O_2 deficit.
    b. a decreased O_2 debt.
    c. a and b
    d. none of the above are correct.

Answer- a

7. The 5 hormones that show a blunted response (decreased secretion) during submaximal exercise are:
    a. insulin, ACTH, cortisol, Growth hormone, thyroid hormone.
    b. ACTH, glycogen, epinephrine, thyroid hormone, growth hormone.
    c. epinephrine, hexokinase, insulin, glucagon, growth hormone.
    d. glucagon, insulin, epinephrine, cortisol, growth hormone.

Answer- d

8. The increased reliance on fat as a fuel as a result of aerobic training is called:
    a. glycolytic adaptation.
    b. glucagon effect.
    c. glycogen sparing effect.
    d. lypolytic increase effect.

Answer- c

9. Which of the following glycolytic enzymes show metabolic adaptations to training?
    a. phosphofructokinase, LDH, PFK, lactase
    b. hexokinase, PFK, glycerolase, ATPase
    c. PFK, LDH, RER, RPE
    d. hexokinase, phosphorylase, PFK, LDH

Answer- d

10. To facilitate metabolic adaptations, the following training cycle should be incorporated:
    a. alternate hard-easy days of training
    b. train hard every day, but reduce training volume in half
    c. train hard 5 days, easy 1 day, and have one entire day off to ensure complete recovery
    d. let the athlete choose intensity of each workout, since they will be better at knowing how their body has recovered

Answer- a

B. Fill in the Blank

1. A continuous aerobic training session performed at a steady-state pace for an extended period of time or distance is called _____ _____ _____.
   Answer- Long Slow Distance Workout

2. A _____ workout is a type of training session named from the Swedish word meaning "speed play," that combines the aerobic demands of a continuous run with the anaerobic demands of sporadic speed intervals.
   Answer- Fartlek

3. An _____ _____ workout is an aerobic and/or anaerobic workout that consists of three elements: a selected work interval (usually a distance), a target time for that distance, and a predetermined recovery period before the next repetition of the work interval.
   Answer- Interval Training

4. The total amount of work done, usually expressed as mileage or load is termed _____ _____.
   Answer- Training Volume

5. A _____ _____ is described as a reduction in training prior to important competitions that is intended to allow the athlete to recover from previous hard training, maintain physiological conditioning, and improve performance.
   Answer- Training Taper

Chapter 13

NUTRITION FOR FITNESS AND ATHLETICS
Outline

I. Introduction

II. Nutrition and Training

    A. Kilocalories

    B. Carbohydrate

    C. Protein

    D. Fat

    E. Vitamins

    F. Minerals

        1. Microminerals

        2. Macrominerals

III. Nutrition for Competition

    A. Carbohydrate Loading (Glycogen Supercompensation)

    B. Pre-event Meal

    C. Feeding During Exercise

    D. Fluid Ingestion During and After Exercise

IV. Eating Disorders

Chapter 13

NUTRITION FOR FITNESS AND ATHLETICS
Suggested Laboratory Activities

1. Have each student complete a three day dietary and activity recall. Analyze the diet for total kcal·day^{-1}, percentages and g·kg^{-1}·day^{-1} of carbohydrate, fat and protein ingested and vitamin and mineral content. Evaluate the adequacy of the diet according to Table 13.1 and the information presented in the chapter. Each student should present recommendations for specific dietary changes as appropriate on the basis of his/her evaluation.

Chapter 13

NUTRITION FOR FITNESS AND ATHLETICS

Review Questions

1. List the goals for nutrition during training and the goals for nutrition during competition. Explain why they are different.

    Pgs. 328-338
    The goals for nutrition during training are: (1) to provide caloric and nutrient requirements, (2) to incorporate nutritional practices that promote good health, (3) to achieve and maintain optimal body composition and playing weight, (4) to promote recovery from training sessions and for physiological adaptations, and (5) to try variations of pre-competition and competition fuel and fluid intake to determine bodily responses. The goals for nutrition and competition are: (1) to ensure adequate fuel supplies in the pre-event time span, (2) to ensure adequate supplies during the event, no matter what the duration, (3) to facilitate temperature regulation by preventing dehydration, (4) to achieve desired weight classifications while maintaining fuel and water supplies, and (5) to avoid gastrointestinal discomfort during competition. Most individuals spend considerably more time training than competing. These daily nutritional practices are critical for general good health and establishing a solid foundation for performance. Food ingestion that might be optimal for performance on a given day could very well be inadequate over the long term. The competition feeding is simply whatever will maximize performance over the time span of the competition.

2. Prepare a table comparing a balanced diet for a sedentary individual and one for an active individual. Include caloric intake, percentages, and grams per kilogram per day recommendations for the major nutrients, as well as similarities or differences in vitamin, mineral, and fluid ingestion.

Table 13.1

	Sedentary Individual	Active Individual
Protein	12-15%; 0.8 g·kg^{-1}·day^{-1}	12-15%; 1.2-2 g·kg^{-1}·day^{-1}
Fat	30% (10% saturated, unsaturated, polyunsaturated)	20-30% (1/3 saturated, unsaturated, polyunsaturated)
CHO	55-58% 4.5 g·kg^{-1}·day^{-1}	58-68% 8-10 g·kg^{-1}·day^{-1}
Vitamins & Minerals	RDA	RDA
Fluid	monitored by thirst	adequate to prevent dehydration

3. Discuss the positive and negative aspects of a high-carbohydrate diet.

Pgs. 329-333

Positive aspects of a high carbohydrate diet- Because high intensity exercise relies on carbohydrate as the primary fuel and lower intensity exercise needs carbohydrate for the complete utilization of fat as a fuel, a ready supply of carbohydrate is necessary for active people. Individuals, however, can only store so much carbohydrate in the form of muscle and liver glycogen. Therefore, a high carbohydrate diet is necessary to replenish used glycogen and avoid fatigue and/or incomplete recovery between training bouts.

Negative aspects of a high carbohydrate diet- Absorption of a large dose of high glycemic carbohydrate results in temporary hyperglycemia and an increased insulin response. Glycogen storage is limited in sedentary and non-endurance trained individuals, and the glycolytic pathway is overloaded. The result is a greater than normal reliance on a side metabolic pathway that converts the glucose to free fatty acids, triglycerides and cholesterol. Absorption of the same amount of low glycemic carbohydrates results in less lipid formation. High blood levels of cholesterol are a risk factor for cardiovascular disease. Endurance athletes appear able to convert high levels of high glycemic carbohydrates into glycogen storage without an elevation of blood lipids. Therefore, this would not be a negative aspect for such individuals.

4. Define glycemic index, and describe how foods are divided into high, moderate and low categories. Using the glycemic index, develop a post-Century bike ride (100 miles) snack to be eaten approximately 30 minutes after the ride, and develop a snack to be eaten during a day of hiking on the Appalachian Trail. Explain your choices.

   Table 13.2, 13.3; Pgs. 331-333
   The glycemic index is a measure that compares the elevation in blood glucose caused by the ingestion of 50 grams of any carbohydrate food with the elevation caused by the ingestion of 50 grams of white bread. White bread has been assigned a glycemic index of 100. The glycemic index is dependent upon the speed at which foods are digested and absorbed. High glycemic foods have a rating of >85, moderate foods have a rating between 60-65, and low glycemic foods have a rating less than 60. Values > 100 are possible.

Post Century Bike Ride Snack	Appalachian Trail Hiking Snack
Should be moderate and high glycemic index foods to cause a fast, high elevation in glucose and insulin for an optimal rate of glycogen resynthesis- Examples- Bagel with jam, sports drink or gel, grapes or raisins, sports bar which includes protein	Selection should be low glycemic foods to maintain a sustained presence of glucose in the system. Examples- Yogurt, apples, sports drink with high fructose content

5. Discuss the situations in which an increase in protein above the RDA is advisable and situations in which such an increase is not advisable.

   Pgs. 333-335
   Situations in which an increase in protein above the RDA is advisable:
   a) activity involving large increase in muscle mass as a primary goal of training
   - Increases in muscle mass and size are accompanied by increases in protein within the muscle fibers. This protein comes from a decrease in endogenous protein breakdown and increased protein synthesis from amino acids. To accommodate the fact these two activities do not precisely balance out and to maintain a positive nitrogen balance, an increase above the RDA is needed.
   b) endurance training
   - Sports anemia my result from protein degradation (in which blood proteins including erythrocytes may be used to increase myoglobin concentration, mitochondrial mass or enzymes) and/or dilution (wherein plasma volume increases but erythrocytes do not). An increased intake of dietary

protein may minimize the destruction of red blood cells, promote their regeneration, and provide protein needed for the other training adaptations to occur. In addition, long duration training and competition results in an increased amino acid oxidation as fuel. Cool temperatures training and females training in the midluteal phases (days 14-21) of the menstrual cycle use more protein as fuel. Finally, additional protein may be needed to avoid overtraining. The use of large amounts of BCAA as fuel leads to increased levels of serotonin which in turn may lead to many of the signs and symptoms of overtraining. Replacement of BCAA may avoid these problems.

c) At the very least, additional protein may be beneficial to ensure repair or any damaged muscle fibers.

Situations in which an increase in protein above the RDA is not advisable:

a) in individuals with pre-existing liver or kidney abnormalities
b) in sedentary individuals. Increased dietary protein in sedentary individuals can lead to increased calcium excretion, suggesting a loss of bone density.

6. Describe a training situation and the theory behind when fat intake can be too low.

Pgs. 335-336
Too little fat in the diet during training can cause a decrement in physiological and performance variables. The theory behind this is that muscle triglycerides are significantly depleted during relatively high-intensity submax exercise. If low concentrations of intramuscular triglycerides are present at the onset of such activity, this leads to a reduced availability of FFA substrate for oxidative metabolism. To compensate, an increased uptake of plasma FFA is necessary, but the rate of delivery to the working muscles may not be sufficient to supply the needed substrate. Thus, just as glycogen can be depleted from the muscle cells and blood borne glucose not be sufficient to offset this, the intramuscular FFA depletion can not be compensated for by blood borne FFA.

7. Compare the theory behind the use of carbohydrate loading for endurance athletes with the theory behind the use of carbohydrates loading for bodybuilders.

Pgs. 339-340
The theory for carbohydrate loading in endurance athletes is that although a high starting level of muscle glycogen will not enable an athlete to perform at a higher intensity, it will allow him/her to maintain a given pace for a longer amount of time. Body builders also participate in carbohydrate loading, but for very different reasons. They have no interest in the energy requirement as does the endurance athlete, however, they are aware that each gram of CHO is stored with 2.7 gram of water. Therefore, if they have a high intake of CHO and restrict themselves from having any fluids, the CHO is supposed to pull the water from within the tissues and away from subcutaneous sites which gives them increased muscle definition. No scientific evidence supports the body builders' theory.

8. Compare the classic and the modified techniques of carbohydrate loading in terms of diet and exercise for endurance athletes. Explain the reasons for the modifications.

Table 13.4; Pgs. 338-340

		Classic	Modified
Diet	Day: -7	mixed diet 50% CHO	50% CHO
	Day: -6	<5% CHO	50% CHO
	Day: -5	< 5% CHO	50% CHO
	Day: -4	< 5% CHO	50% CHO
	Day: -3	80-90% CHO	70% CHO
	Day: -2	80-90% CHO	70% CHO
	Day: -1	80-90% CHO	70% CHO
	competition	High CHO pre-event	High CHO pre-event
Exercise	Day-7	exercise to exhaustion	90 min 75% VO2max
	Day: -6	90-120 min 65-85% VO_2max	same as above
	Day: -5	same as above	40 min 75% VO_2max
	Day: -4	same as above	same as above
	Day: -3	rest	20 min 75% VO_2max
	Day: -2	rest	same as above
	Day: -1	rest	rest
	competition	event	event

Reasons for the modifications to the classic carbohydrate loading technique:
a) The ingestion of only 5% CHO for 3 days leads to an unhealthy level of fat intake.
b) Fat burns in the flame of CHO. With so little CHO, the ingested fat is incompletely metabolized and ketosis occurs.
c) Hypoglycemia can occur with such low CHO ingestion leading to fatigue, restlessness, mental disturbances, irritability and

weakness. Hard training is difficult if not impossible to maintain.
- d) When the switch is made to 80-90% CHO the individual can feel stiff and heavy due to water retention. Weight gain can equal 1-2 kg.
- e) Neither the exhaustive glycogen depletion exercise nor the 3 days of high protein, high fat diet are needed to maximize muscle glycogen storage.

a-d lead to psychological and physiological "down" feeling.

9. Prepare a table of a comprehensive fluid and nutrient intake for preevent, during-the-event, and postevent diets for a football player and a triathlete.

Table 13.5; Pgs. 340-343

	Football	**Triathlete**
Pre-event	Fluid: ingestion 3-4 hr, 30 min Food: light balance meal, high %CHO	Fluid: ingestion 3-4 hr, 30 min Food: 200-500kcal, 0-5 minutes prior to competition 50-100 g CHO
Event	Water as desired	Fluid ingestion CHO (opt) 30-60 g·hr^{-1}, [6-10%] CHO, some Na
Post-event	Fluid ingestion	Fluid ingestion CHO 50-100g, some Na

10. Define and list the characteristics of anorexia nervosa, bulimia nervosa, and anorexia athletica.

Table 13.6; Pgs. 343-344

Anorexia Nervosa	Bulimia Nervosa	Anorexia Athletica
• Refusal to maintain body weight above that considered normal for height and age; marked self-induced weight loss • Intense fear of weight gain or becoming fat despite being underweight • Endocrine changes manifested by amenorrhea in females and loss of sexual interest and potency in males	• Recurrent episodes of binge eating • Purging or compensating for bingeing by self-induced vomiting, use of diuretics or laxatives, vigorous exercise, and strict food restriction or fasting • Exhibiting bingeing or inappropriate compensatory behavior at least twice a week for three months • Unrealistic appraisal of body weight and shape	• Weight loss; > 5% below normal for age and height • Absence of medical disorder to explain weight loss • Excess feat of becoming fat • Food intake < 1200 kcal·day^{-1} • Delayed puberty • Primary or secondary amenorrhea or oligomenorrhea • Binge eating that is not high in calories • Purging • Gastrointestinal complaints • Distorted body image • Compulsive exercise in addition to normal needed training

11. Identify the risk factors for developing an eating disorder. Prepare a set of guidelines that might be useful in counteracting these risk factors or dealing with the disorder early in its progression

    Pgs. 344-347
    Risk factors for eating disorders include: dieting at an early age, especially if recommended by a coach; unsupervised dieting given by someone who is untrained in proper nutrition; lack of acceptance of pubertal change; early sport-specific training, body type has a huge influence on sports, outgrowing a selected sport can be devastating; large increase in training volume accompanied by significant weight loss; and traumatic events. Guidelines to help prevent these risk factors include: encourage children to try a variety of sports; identify realistic, healthy weight goals; monitor their weight and body composition to detect continued and unwanted weight losses; provide nutritional guidance; provide realist training program; avoid overtraining and injury; provide a supportive atmosphere for accepting pubertal changes; be aware of symptoms of eating disorders; and seek professional help if there is any suspicion of an eating disorder. Students may suggest other good strategies.

Chapter 13

NUTRITION FOR FITNESS AND ATHLETICS
Exam Questions

A. Multiple Choice

1. When a runner hits the wall, this means that (s)he:
   a. has exceeded O_2 capacity and can no longer tolerate the lactic acid.
   b. has reached anaerobic threshold and must slow down.
   c. has exhausted his/her muscle glycogen supply and must utilize fatty acids as the major fuel.
   d. has exceeded the limits of his sympathetic nervous system and the parasympathetic is regaining control.

Answer- c

2. What is the normal RDA for an adult for carbohydrate? What is recommended for an athlete training for an endurance event?
   a. $2 \text{ g·kg}^{-1}\text{·day}^{-1}$; $4.5 \text{ g·kg}^{-1}\text{·day}^{-1}$
   b. $4.5 \text{ g·kg}^{-1}\text{·day}^{-1}$; $8\text{-}10 \text{ g·kg}^{-1}\text{·day}^{-1}$
   c. $8\text{-}10 \text{ g·kg}^{-1}\text{·day}^{-1}$; $12\text{-}15 \text{ g·kg}^{-1}\text{·day}^{-1}$
   d. $12\text{-}15 \text{ g·kg}^{-1}\text{·day}^{-1}$; $20\text{-}30 \text{ g·kg}^{-1}\text{·day}^{-1}$

Answer- b

3. The glycemic index:
   a. is dependent upon whether a carbohydrate is simple or complex; simple sugars have a high glycemic index while complex carbohydrates have a low glycemic index.
   b. is dependent upon the speed at which carbohydrates are digested and absorbed; foods with a high glycemic index cause a fast, high elevation in glucose and insulin whereas foods with a low glycemic index cause a slower rise in both.
   c. high glycemic foods such as most fruits, legumes and dairy products are preferred for glycogen resynthesis.
   d. a, b, and c are correct.

Answer- b

4. The rate at which an ingested fluid enters the body's supply is dependent upon four factors. Which of the following is not a true factor?
   a. Gastric emptying rate decreases as the caloric content of the ingested fluid increases.
   b. Sodium greatly decreases intestinal fluid absorption over plain water.
   c. The amount of fluid emptied from the stomach is large immediately after drinking and then slows down as the volume decreases.
   d. The gastric emptying rate of hot and cold fluids are similar.

Answer- b

5. Which of the following is not true regarding glycogen resynthesis?
   a. Carbohydrate ingestion (50-100g) should begin as soon after a workout or competition as is practical (15-30 min).
   b. Resynthesis occurs at about 5-6% per hour when eating approximately 50g of CHO every 2 hours.
   c. Liquid CHO is as effective as solid CHO
   d. Storage of liver and muscle glycogen is maximized after a muscle is exhausted by eccentric muscle work.

Answer- d

6. Which of the following is not true regarding carbohydrate/electrolyte/fluid replacement?
   a. If an event is shorter than 30 minutes, the preferred beverage is plain water.
   b. If the event is between 1 and 2 hours or takes place in high heat and humidity, the CHO concentration should be 2.5-8% and the sodium content 30-110 mg.
   c. If the event is between 2 and 4 hours in moderate environmental conditions, the CHO concentration should be 6-10% and the sodium concentration 30-110 mg.
   d. If the event is longer than 4 hours, the ingestion of any concentration of CHO and sodium can lead to "water intoxication" (hyponatremia).

Answer- d

7. What is the normal daily requirement of protein? What is recommended for an athlete involved in weight training?
   a. $0.6 \text{ g·kg}^{-1}\text{·day}^{-1}$; $0.8\text{-}1.1 \text{ g·kg}^{-1}\text{·day}^{-1}$
   b. $0.8 \text{ g·kg}^{-1}\text{·day}^{-1}$; $1.2\text{-}2.0 \text{ g·kg}^{-1}\text{·day}^{-1}$
   c. $1.2 \text{ g·kg}^{-1}\text{·day}^{-1}$; $1.2\text{-}2.0 \text{ g·kg}^{-1}\text{·day}^{-1}$
   d. $0.8 \text{ g·kg}^{-1}\text{·day}^{-1}$; $2.5\text{-}3.7 \text{ g·kg}^{-1}\text{·day}^{-1}$

Answer- b

8. A high protein diet (in excess of 15% PRO):
    a. is necessary for athletes doing heavy resistance training.
    b. is recommended for athletes competing at sprint and middle distances.
    c. is important when athletes reduce the level of training to prevent muscle atrophy.
    d. increases the excretion of calcium which may be detrimental to amenorrheic athletes.

Answer- d

9. An individual exhibits the following symptoms:
    - Body weight more than 5% below normal for age and height without medical cause
    - Food intake of <1200 kcal·day^{-1}
    - Delayed puberty
    - Bingeing of non-calorically dense foods followed by purging
    - Compulsive exercise in excess of fitness or training needs

    These are indicative of:
    a. anorexia nervosa
    b. bulimia nervosa
    c. anorexia athletica
    d. normal accepted behavior

Answer- c

10. New sports bars (PR Bar and Beta Bar) use the 40-30-30 ratio of CHO, protein, and fat. The rationale for the use of these bars prior to exercise would be:
    a. With the increase in glucagon release, and inhibition of insulin release, more fat will be used as fuel during exercise.
    b. With the higher levels of protein, damage to the muscle cells will be reduced.
    c. There will be more available BCAA to facilitate the levels of serotonin to reduce muscle fatigue.
    d. none of the above are correct.

Answer-a

Fill in the Blank

1. _____ _____ is a measure that compares the elevation in blood glucose caused by the ingestion of 50 g of any carbohydrate food with the elevation caused by the ingestion of 50 g of white bread.

    Answer- Glycemic Index

2. A transient decrease in red blood cells and hemoglobin levels (grams per deciliter of blood)Vitamins, Organic substances of plant or animal origin which are essential for normal growth, development, metabolic processes, and energy transformations is called _____ _____.

   Answer- Sports Anemia

3. Elements not of animal or plant origin which are essential constituents of all cells and of many functions in the body are called _____.
   Answer- Minerals

4. _____ _____ is a process of nutritional modification that results in an additional storage of glycogen in muscle fiber that can be approximately three to four times the normal levels.
   Answer- Carbohydrate Loading (Glycogen Supercompensation)

5. An eating disorder characterized by marked self-induced weight loss accompanied by an intense fear of fatness and reproductive hormonal changes is called _____ _____.

   Answer- Anorexia Nervosa

6. An eating disorder marked by an unrealistic appraisal of body weight and/or shape that is manifested by alternating bingeing and purging behavior is called _____ _____.

   Answer- Bulimia Nervosa

7. An eating disorder occurring primarily in young, female athletes that is characterized by a food intake less than that required to support the training regimen and by body weight no more than 95% of normal is called _____ _____.
   Answer- Anorexia Athletica

Chapter 14

BODY COMPOSITION: DETERMINATION AND IMPORTANCE
Outline

I. Introduction

II. Body Composition Assessment

    A. Laboratory Techniques

        1. Hydrostatic (Underwater) Weighing: Densitometry

        2. Densitometry: Children and Adolescents, and the Elderly

    B. Field Tests of Body Composition

        1. Skinfolds

        2. Bioelectrical Impedance (Impedance Plethysmography)

        3. Height and Weight

        4. Body Mass Index

III. Overweight and Obesity

    A. What Happens to Adipose Cells in Obesity? The Cellular Basis of Obesity

    B. Fat Distribution Patterns

    C. Waist-to-Hip Ratio

    D. Health Risks of Overweight and Obesity

        1. Cardiovascular Disease

        2. Hypertension (High Blood Pressure)

        3. Gallbladder Disease and Hypercholesterolemia (High Cholesterol)

        4. Diabetes Mellitus

        5. Cancer

        6. Miscellaneous Disorders

IV. Heredity and Body Composition

Chapter 14

BODY COMPOSITION: DETERMINATION AND IMPORTANCE
Suggested Laboratory Activities

1. Determine body composition by:
   - hydrostatic weighing
   - bioelectrical impedance
   - skinfolds

   Compare and contrast the results.

2. Determine body composition by hydrostatic weighing for as many class members as possible. Have each compute his/her ideal weight based on healthy, realistic percent fat goals.

3. Have each student determine his/her body mass index (BMI) and evaluate it against the standards presented in Table 14.4 and Figure 14.6.

4. Have each student determine his/her waist-to-hip ratio and evaluate it against the standards presented on pg. 369.

Chapter 14

BODY COMPOSITION: DETERMINATION AND IMPORTANCE
Review Questions

1. Define denstiometry. Relate denstiometry to hydrostatic weighing.

    Pgs. 353-357
    Densitometry is the measurement of mass per unit of volume. Whole body denstiometry is the foundation of hydrostatic weighing. It is based on dividing the body into fat and fat-free mass (or fat-free weight). Hydrostatic weighing determines body density (D_B), defined as mass (M) or weight (wt) divided by volume (V_G) according to the formula:

    $$D_B = \frac{M_A}{\frac{(M_A - M_W)}{D_W} - (RV + V_B)}$$

    The numerator, mass, is obtained by weighing the individual. The denominator, volume, is based on Archimedes' principle. Archimedes principle states that a submerged object experiences an upward buoyant force equal to the weight or the volume of fluid displace by the object. This means that the volume of any object, including the human body, can be measured by determining the weight lost by complete submersion underwater. The weight loss ($M_A - M_W$) is corrected for the density of the water, residual volume and intestinal gas.

2. Explain the assumptions that must be met in order for hydrostatic weighing to be accurate. What variations in these basic assumptions occur in children, adolescents, and the elderly? State two practical applications of this information.

    Pgs. 354, 357-359
    The assumptions that need to be met in order to accurately calculate %BF in hydrostatic weighing are: (a) the densities of the fat and fat free weight are known and additive; (b) the densities of water,

mineral and protein which make up the FFW are known and relatively constant from individual to individual; (c) the percentage of each fat free component is relatively stable from individual to individual; and (d) the individual being evaluated differs only from the assumptions of the equation being used in the amount of storage fat. Fat free weight for adults is assumed to be composed of 73% water, 20% protein and 7% minerals for an overall density of 1.1 $g \cdot cc^{-1}$. While the percentage of protein is relatively stable over the growth years the other values are not. The percentage of water in FFW decreases from 77-78% at ages 7-9 to 73% at age 20 in a steady but slightly curvilinear fashion. Conversely, the mineral content increases from approximately 5% at ages 7-9 to the 7% at age 20. The result of these changes is that body density also increases in a curvilinear fashion from approximately 1.08 to 1.10 $g \cdot cc^{-1}$ for adult males and to 1.095 $g \cdot cc^{-1}$ for adult females. While the values for boys and girls change in the same direction, girls always have a higher water content (and percentage) and lower mineral content (and percentage). In the elderly, osteoporosis can lead to a loss of bone mineral.

Practical applications:
a) Adult equations for determining percent body fat from body density cannot be used for children and adolescents.
b) Separate equations are needed for boys and girls.
c) Equations developed on young and middle aged adults may overestimate percent body fat in the elderly.

3. List and identify the strengths and weaknesses of the field estimates of overweight and obesity. Which techniques would you select to use in a field setting? Explain why.

Pgs. 359-264

Skinfolds Strengths: the accuracy in the prediction of %BF is approximately 3-5% in comparison to hydrostatic weighing. This is specific to sex and age. Weaknesses: it is a technical skill subjected to human error and if measured incorrectly, can result in large prediction errors.

Bioelectrical Impedance Strengths: ease at which it can be conducted, easy to use, consistent under standard conditions. Weaknesses: because it actually measures total body water, it is highly dependent upon the maintenance of a normal level of hydration. It is also dependent upon both ambient and skin temperatures. Any change in the above variables will alter the reading of % BF. Accuracy is limited to individual not the extremes of leanness of fatness.

Height-Weight Strengths: ease of measurement, normative and evaluative tables are readily available. Weaknesses: based on an insurance group and not a random sample; people with heart disease, cancer and/or diabetes were excluded; only body weights or time of purchases not death were included; many values were self reported; no definition of frame size, and does not provide information of body composition.

Body Mass Index Strengths: ease of determination, uses only height and weight. It is highly correlated with mortality. Weaknesses: there is a considerate amount of error in using BMI as an estimate of body adiposity.

Students should select skinfolds because of its high correlation with hydrostatic weighing.

4. Compare the accuracy of % BF determined by skinfolds and bioelectrical impedance with % BF determined by hydrostatic weighting.

   Pgs. 360, 262
   The accuracy of both skinfold and BIA prediction of %body fat is approximately 3-5% compared with under water weighing.

5. Compare and contrast the % BF, % BF distribution, and patterns of fat distribution between males and females.

   Tables 14.2, 14.5; Figure 14.7; Pgs. 364-369
   %BF: Prior to puberty there is very little sex difference. After puberty, male values drop while female values rise slowly. After age 30, both male and female values rise with female values rising more than male values. Thus, throughout adulthood female %BF exceeds male %BF by average. Females have ~50% more fat cells than males.

   %BF distribution: Females have similar (12% vs. 15-18%) amounts of storage fat to males. Likewise the percentage of body fat in the abdominal thoracic cavity (2% vs. 1%), within muscles (1% vs. 1%) and between muscles (6% vs. 5%) is similar between the sexes. However, the subcutaneous storage portion is twice as high for females as males (9% vs. 4%) and essential fat is three to four times as high (9-12 vs. 3%).

   Patterns of fat distribution: Most females store fat in the gynoid pattern, while most males store fat in the android pattern. The gynoid pattern is characterized by fat storage in the lower part of the body (thighs and buttocks) with the largest quantity being stored subcutaneously. The android pattern is characterized by fat storage in the upper body (nape of the neck, shoulders and abdomen) with the largest quantity being stored internally.

6. Differentiate between overweight and obesity.

> **Table 14.4; Pg. 364**
> Obesity is defined as the pathological condition in which an individual possess an excess of body fat the represents a significant health risk; males >25%, females >32%. Overweight is defined as a situation in which an individual carries an excess (10 - 20%) of body weight in relation to height or stature; it indicates mild or moderate health risks. The difference is obesity is defined in terms of body composition (%BF) while overweight does not consider body composition, although equivalent values are available. Obesity carries a more significant health risk.

7. What happens to adipose cells as an individual becomes overweight and then obese?

> **Pgs. 364-367**
> Adipocytes first change in size to accommodate higher amounts of stored triglycerides. Adipocytes can change in size about tenfold. Once the upper limit of fat storage by hypertrophy is approached (~30 kg of fat), fat cell hyperplasia occurs. This means new adipocytes develop from immature precursor cells. Adipocytes themselves do not divide and multiply. Once created these fat cells are not naturally reduced.

8. List and briefly discuss the health risks of being overweight or obese.

> **Pgs. 369-370**
> Overweight individuals incur mild to moderate health risks. Obese individuals incur high risk of major diseases. These health/disease risks include:
> a) *cardiovascular disease*- Evidence from the Framingham study indicates that overweight or obesity is a significant predictor of cardiovascular disease independent of age, cholesterol, systolic blood pressure, cigarette smoking, and glucose tolerance. The risk is greater for these who become obese early in life rather than old age and for those who store fat in the android rather than the gynoid pattern.
> b) *hypertension*- The relationship between hypertension and overweight/obesity is direct as is the relationship between hypertension and CHD.
> c) *gallbladder disease*- Excess body weight/fat increases cholesterol production. The bile (stored in the gallbladder) of overweight/obese individuals is more saturated with cholesterol

than that of non-obese individuals. The result is an increased incidence of gallbladder disease.

    d) *diabetes mellitus*- Overweight/obesity causes a deterioration in glucose tolerance and aggravates the appearance of diabetes.

    e) *cancer*- Overweight/obese males are particularly susceptible to prostate and colorectal cancer. Overweight/obese females are particularly susceptible to breast, cervical, endometrial uterine and ovarian cancer. High levels of estrogen formed in adipose tissue is the link for females.

9. Debate the importance of heredity in body composition.

Pgs. 370-371
In very few individuals (1 in 25,000), both obesity and the localization of fat deposition are determined solely by genetics. For the vast majority of individuals, much if not most (45-65%) of the variance in body composition is not genetic. The storage of internal fat is probably influenced more by genetics than is the storage of subcutaneous fat. The tendency to gain fat mass or fat-free mass (nutrient partitioning) is genetic.

Chapter 14

BODY COMPOSITION: DETERMINATION AND IMPORTANCE
Exam Questions

A. Multiple Choice

1. In determining body density/percent body fat:
   a. hydrostatic (underwater) weighing is considered the criterion measure and assumes that the body is divided into two compartments, fat and fat free weight.
   b. the accuracy of skinfold prediction is approximately 3-5% when compared to underwater weighing.
   c. by bioelectrical impedance, total body water is actually measured from the flow of an electrical current, but the accuracy is no better than for skinfolds.
   d. a, b, and c are correct

   Answer- d

2. Given the following information, calculate the individual's BMI.
   Sex = M   Height = 5'8"
   Weight = 165 lbs Age = 42 yr.
   a. 25.2
   b. 43.4
   c. 24.3
   d. 33.3

   Answer- a

3. The subject in the above problem:
   a. has an acceptable BMI.
   b. has a BMI that is too high, indicating an excess mortality.
   c. has a BMI that is too low, indicating an excess mortality.
   d. has no BMI that can be calculated with the given information.

   Answer- a

4. Cellulite:
   a. is difficult to mobilize. Female sex specific fat depots of the thigh and hips.
   b. appears when enlarged adipocytes cause a bulging between the fibrous connective tissue strands.
   c. can be detected by its dimply, waffled appearance but is otherwise not physiologically special.
   d. a, b, and c are correct
   e. b and c are correct

Answer- e

5. When an adult gains weight:
   a. increasing levels of fat are first stored by fat cell hypertrophy and then through hyperplasia.
   b. (s)he changes his or her basic body shape, i.e. from gynoid to cubic, or android to gynoid, etc.
   c. hyperplasia is achieved by cell division of existing fat cells which then hypertrophy and fill.
   d. a, b, and c are correct

Answer- a

6. Essential % body fat and obese % body fat which carries a significant health risk for male and female, respectively, are:
   a. 11% essential, >32% risk; 11% essential, >26% risk
   b. 11% essential, 12-18% risk; 3% essential, >32% risk
   c. 3% essential, 19-24% risk; 11% essential, >26-31% risk
   d. 3% essential, >25% risk; 11% essential, >32% risk

Answer- d

7. Humans distribute fat in three basic patterns: the android, gynoid, and intermediate or cubic.
   a. The android pattern, found primarily in males, is characterized by upper body, internal abdominal storage before subcutaneous sites are loaded.
   b. The gynoid pattern, found primarily in females, differs from the android only in that the storage occurs primarily in the hip and thigh region.
   c. The android pattern tends to be hard and misinterpreted as superior musculature while the gynoid storage tends to be soft and jiggly.
   d. a, b, and c are correct.
   e. a and c are correct.

Answer- e

8. The health risks associated with obesity include, but are not necessarily limited to:
   a. cardiovascular disease, especially for those possessing the android obese pattern.
   b. gall bladder disease, especially linked with hypercholesteremia.
   c. Diabetes Mellitus, especially if adult onset.
   d. a, b, and c are correct.

Answer- d

9. LBM represents:
   i. lowest basal metabolism
   j. lean body mass
   k. less body mass
   l. lower body mass

Answer- b

10. The accuracy of skinfold measurements (assuming a trained professional takes the measurement) when compared to under water weighing is:
   j. 3-5%
   k. <1%
   l. 10%
   m. 5-10%

Answer- a

B. Fill in the Blank

1. _____ _____ is a criterion measure for determining body composition through the calculation of body density.
   Answer- Hydrostatic Weighing

2. _____ _____ is the principle that a partially or fully submerged object will experience an upward buoyant force equal to the weight or the volume of fluid displaced by the object.
   Answer- Archimedes' Principle

3. The measurement of mass per unit volume is called _____.
   Answer- Densitometry

4. The weight of body tissue excluding extractable fat is called _____ _____.
   Answer- Fat-Free Weight

5. The partitioning of body mass into fat-free mass (weight or percentage) and fat mass (weight or percentage) is called _____ _____.
   Answer- Body composition

6. _____ is the double thickness of skin plus the adipose tissue between the parallel layers of skin.
Answer- Skinfolds

7. _____ is the growth in a tissue or organ through an increase in the number of cells.
Answer- Hyperplasia

Chapter 15

BODY COMPOSITION AND WEIGHT CONTROL

Outline

I. The Caloric Balance Equation

   A. Food Ingested

      1. Impact of Diet on Food Intake

      2. Impact of Exercise and Exercise Training on Food Intake

   B. Resting or Basal Metabolism

      1. The Impact of Diet on Resting Metabolic Rate

      2. The Impact of Exercise on Resting Metabolic Rate

      3. Exercise Training and Resting Metabolic Rate

      4. Weight Cycling

   C. Thermogenesis

      1. The Impact of Diet on the Thermic Effect of a Meal

      2. The Impact of Exercise on the Thermic Effect of a Meal

      3. Exercises Training and the Thermic Effect of a Meal

   D. The Impact of Diet, Exercise and Exercise Training on Energy Expenditure

   E. The Effect of Diet, Exercise Training, and Diet Plus Exercise Training on Body Composition and Weight

      1. The Effects of Diet on Body Composition and Weight

      2. The Effects of Exercise Training on Body Composition and Weight

      3. The Effects of Diet Plus Exercise Training on Body Composition and Weight

II. Applications of the Training Principles for Weight and Body Composition Loss and/or Control

   A. Specificity

    B. Overload

    C. Adaptation

    D. Progression

    E. Individualization

    F. Retrogression/Plateau/Reversibility

    G. Maintenance

III. Making Weight for Sport

Chapter 15

BODY COMPOSITION AND WEIGHT CONTROL

Suggested Laboratory Activities

1. Using the metabolic cart:
   - Measure the basal or resting metabolic rate of one or more students using oxygen consumption techniques. Express the results in kcal·day^{-1}, kcal·m^{-2}·hr^{-1}, and mL·kg·$^{-1}$min^{-1}. Compare and contrast the results with the definition for one MET.
   - Have students compute their basal or resting metabolic rates using the equations in Table 15.2.
   - Compare and contrast the measure versus calculated metabolic rates.
   - Compare and contrast the measured metabolic rates between:
     ⇒ a male and a female of equal training status.
     ⇒ an aerobically trained versus an untrained individual of the same sex and approximate body size.
     ⇒ a dynamic resistance trained versus an untrained individual of the same sex and approximate body size.

2. Have students complete a 24 hour dietary recall under two conditions:
   - time zero = a moderate intensity 45 minute workout of the student's choosing
   - same time of day as above, but no exercise is to occur in the following 24 hour period

   Calculate the caloric intake for both days and compare and contrast the results.

3. Measure the thermic effect of a meal alone and compare and contrast these results with the thermic effect of an exercise bout either before or after the same meal in the same individual.

4. Use the three day dietary and activity recall completed for Chapter 13 and the basal or resting metabolic rate obtained in this chapter. Have each student determine his/her caloric balance and interpret it with regard to weight maintenance, weight loss, or weight gain.

Chapter 15

BODY COMPOSITION AND WEIGHT CONTROL

Review Questions

1. State the caloric balance equation, and relate it to the first law of thermodynamics. Define and explain the components of the caloric balance equation.

   Pg. 376
   Caloric Balance = + food ingested
   - basal (resting) metabolic rate (kcal)
   - thermogenesis (kcal)
   - work or exercise metabolism (kcal)
   - energy excreted in waste products (kcal)

   The *caloric balance* equation quantifies the first law of thermodynamics. Potential chemical energy in the form of food is converted into mechanical energy, heat energy or other chemical energy and either used, stored or dissipated as heat or excretion. Energy is neither created nor destroyed, but simply changed in form. *Basal metabolic rate* is the level of energy required to sustain the body's vital functions in the waking state when the individual is in a fasted condition, at normal body and room temperature, and without psychological stress. Resting metabolic rate is the energy expenditure while an individual is resting quietly in a supine position. The liver is the largest consumer of energy at rest (29-32%), followed by the brain (19-21%), muscles (18%), heart (10%), lungs (9%), and kidneys (7%). The energy is used to maintain muscle tone, fuel ion pumps, synthesize and degrade cellular constituents, conduct electrical impulses, and secrete hormones and other substances.

   Thermogenesis is the production of heat. An increased energy expenditure occurs after the ingestion of food. Some of this energy is due to digestion, absorption, assimilation, and synthesis of foodstuffs. The rest simply appears as heat. The mechanism of thermogenesis is unknown but it has been linked to an uncoupling of oxidative phosphorylation and/or brown adipose tissue activity.

Work or exercise metabolism is simply energy expended in activities above the resting level.
Energy excreted in waste products is insignificant and rarely quantified. Such energy is lost to the body but not the universe.

2. Discuss the impact of dietary restriction on the components of the caloric balance equation.

Table 15.3; Pgs. 377-381, 384, 385

Caloric Balance Factor	Diet
Food ingested (+)	By definition, a reduction occurs
BMR and/or RMR (-)	Severe caloric restriction causes a 10-20% decrease; weight cycling does not decrease
Thermogenesis (-)	Decreases because fewer calories are being ingested; dependent on composition of meals
Work or exercise expenditure (-)	If calories are insufficient, may voluntarily do less exercise; but no direct effect on caloric cost

3. Discuss the impact of exercise on the components of the caloric balance equation.

Table 15.3; Pgs. 381-385

Caloric Balance Factor	Exercise
Food ingested (+)	No clearly established effect; appetite does not decrease
BMR and/or RMR (-)	Unchanged per se but metabolic rate postexercise remains elevated
Thermogenesis (-)	No consistent additive effect in either a sequence of food-exercise or exercise food
Work or exercise expenditure (-)	By definition, an increase occurs

4. Discuss the impact of exercise training on the components of the caloric balance equation.

Table 15.3; Pgs. 381-385

Caloric Balance Factor	Exercise Training
Food ingested (+)	Energy intake increases (highly trained and lean individuals) or remains constant (untrained and obese individuals); when training ceases, food intake spontaneously decreases but does not match the decrease in expenditure
BMR and/or RMR (-)	No consistent effect is evident
Thermogenesis (-)	Inverted U response, dependent on fitness level; moderate levels of fitness and training increase thermogenesis; high levels of fitness decrease thermogenesis
Work or exercise expenditure (-)	A cumulative increase occurs

5. Compare and contrast the effects of diet alone, exercise alone, and diet and exercise combined on body weight and composition control.

Figures 15.3, 15.5, 15.6; Pgs. 385-391

	Compare	Contrast
Diet	weight/fat is lost if caloric deficit is achieved, majority of early loss is water	highest loss of FFW (LBM), difficult to maintain loss
Exercise	weight/fat is lost if caloric deficit is achieved, majority of early loss is water	FFW (LBM) loss is minimized, maybe maintained or gained. Maintenance of weight loss best through exercise training. Increased health/fitness is added benefit
Diet + Exercise	weight/fat is lost if caloric deficit is achieved, majority of early loss is water	body weight is not lost faster than either individually, but FFW (LBM) is maintained. Can eat more calories and make a better nutrient balance and still achieve loss than if only diet. Best for long term change.

6. List the training principles. Explain how each should be specifically applied for body weight or body composition control or maintenance.

Pgs. 391-395
- *Specificity* - Achieve a caloric deficit of 250-500 kcal·day^{-1} by a combination of dietary restriction, aerobic endurance exercise (3-5 days·week^{-1}) and/or dynamic resistance training (2-3 days·week^{-1})
- *Overload* - Emphasize total number of calories expended in exercise rather than intensity if individuals are initially unfit to increase exercise tolerance. Any combination of frequency, duration and intensity of exercise that will obtain a caloric deficit and be tolerated by the individual is acceptable. Use net, not gross, caloric values when calculating exercise energy expenditure.
- *Adaptation* - Emphasize slow long term weight loss because the proportion of body fat loss is greater after several weeks. Adaptation will be seen as weight loss and dimension changes.
- *Progression* - The greatest progression should be made in the amount of calories that can be expended in exercise. When the amount of calories expended increases, the food intake can either remain the same (increasing the deficit) or match the increase (maintain the original deficit).
- *Individualization* - Do a RMR, nutrient and caloric intake analysis, and energy expenditure analysis on each individual. Base the diet and exercise program on these results.
- *Plateau/Retrogression/Reversibility* - Weight loss is unequal being fastest in the early stages. Reverting to old habits of food intake and a sedentary lifestyle will result in regaining the lost weight/fat.
- *Maintenance* - The key is exercise training.

7. Defend or refute the following statements, using evidence provided in this chapter.

Pgs. 382-383
(a) *Weight cycling makes subsequent weight loss physiologically more difficult.*
Refute- the study by Blackburn et al that found that prior weight loss made subsequent weight loss harder had flaws; the subjects were older during the second weight loss sequence and age decreases in RMR; there was less adherence to the diet during the second weight loss cycle. Studies by Beeson et al., vanDale et al., and Wadden et al., found no relationship between weight loss cycles and the subsequent rate or amount of weight loss in other cycles.

Pg. 377, 390

(b) The most important reason to add exercise or exercise training to a weight loss or maintenance program is that exercise decreases appetite.

Refute- Neither a transient reduction nor an increase in energy intake immediately following a single bout of exercise has been established in humans. In one study despite a subjective rating of lower appetite after exercise, food intake for the next two days was not affected. Energy intake generally increases or remains unchanged in response to exercise training.

Pg. 384

(c) If food is eaten near the time of exercise (either directly prior to or after), the thermic response is potentiated (made more effective), so that more calories are burned and weight is lost faster.

Refute- Evidence for the potentiation of the thermic effect of food plus exercise is confusing. No clear pattern has emerged from the available studies as to when the effect appears to be additive and when it is not.

Pgs. 381-382

(d) The maintenance of, increase in, or decrease in, resting metabolic rate depends on the maintenance or change in lean body mass.

Refute- Some studies have shown that trained individuals exhibit higher RMRs than sedentary individuals or that training programs bring about an increase in RMR, but others have not. An occasional study has even shown a decrease in RMR when exercise training was added to severe caloric restriction. When subjects were matched by FFW in one study, the trained individuals still had a higher RMR than the untrained despite similar lean mass amounts. Since muscle accounts for only 18% of RMR this is not too surprising. Other studies have shown the RMR increases with the addition of exercise much sooner than any body composition changes could have occurred. RMR is highly related to FFW but not entirely dependent upon it. One study involving resistance training showed both an increase in RMR and FFW. However, the increase in RMR remained significant even when expressed per kilogram of FFW. The RMR increase maybe linked to increased basal sympathetic nervous system activity.

Pg. 393

(e) To lose fat, burn fat by doing long-duration, low-intensity exercise.

Refute- Although it is true that fat is the dominant fuel in long-duration, low-intensity exercise, the important factor in weight loss is to establish a caloric deficit no matter which fuel is being used. The study by Ballor et al., contrasted a low intensity training group that expended 283 kcal per session (66% fat) with a high intensity group that expended 260 kcal per session (26% fat). Both groups lost equal amounts of percent body fat.

8. Prepare a set of weight control guidelines for a jockey.

Pgs. 395-396

Have body composition assessed during the off season. Set as a goal a %BF not less than 5% and not requiring more than a 7% total weight loss. Achieve the desired %BF during the off season and pre-season by a combination of dietary restriction, aerobic endurance and dynamic resistance training. Maintain the %BF during the season by exercise. Avoid weight cycling if possible.

Chapter 15

BODY COMPOSITION AND WEIGHT CONTROL
Exam Questions

A. Multiple Choice

1. The relationship between exercise/exercise training and food intake is such that:
   a. a transient reduction in energy intake immediately following a single bout of activity has been clearly established.
   b. highly trained athletes and lean individuals usually decrease their energy intake in response to increased training loads.
   c. athletes and/or trained individuals generally eat more than untrained individuals with the possible exception of those in aesthetic sports (gymnasts, dancers, etc.).
   d. when chronic exercise training ceases, energy intake in humans spontaneously reduces to match the reduced energy expenditure.

   Answer- c

2. Resting metabolic rate:
   a. is lower for the obese than that of a normal weight individual of the same age, sex, and height.
   b. decreases at any given body weight for each 1% increase in body fat.
   c. increases and decreases with a lowering or raising, respectively, of body core temperature.
   d. averages between 1500 and 1800 kcal·d^{-1} for adult females and 1200 and 1450 kcal·d^{-1} for adult males.

   Answer- b

3. The relationship between diet, exercise, and exercise training and resting metabolic rate is such that:
   a. severe caloric restriction decreases resting metabolic rate.
   b. RMR itself is elevated during exercise, in the recovery from exercise (EPOC), and permanently as a result of exercise training.
   c. the effect of exercise training on RMR is not totally dependent on muscle mass but may also be linked to other factors such as sympathetic nervous activity.
   d. a, b, and c are correct
   e. a and c are correct

   Answer- e

4. Weight cycling:
   a. slows down the resting metabolic rate.
   b. increases the difficulty of subsequent weight loss.
   c. enhances abdominal fat deposition.
   d. does not adversely affect either body fat distribution or body composition.

Answer- d

5. The impact of diet, exercise and exercise training on the thermic effect of a meal is that:
   a. carbohydrates and fat cause a greater thermic response than proteins.
   b. exercise in close proximity to eating (either before or after) consistently increases the thermic effect of the meal (TEM)
   c. moderately trained individuals show an increase in the TEM, but highly trained individuals do not.
   d. a, b, and c are correct
   e. b and c are correct

Answer- c

6. If an individual elects to lose weight by caloric restriction alone:
   a. both body fat and fat free mass will be lost.
   b. during the first several days the majority of the weight loss is water.
   c. restricting water intake while dieting causes a higher proportion of water, not a lower proportion, to be lost.
   d. a, b, and c are correct

Answer- d

7. When using exercise to lose body weight it must be remembered that:
   a. the key to weight and fat loss is the achievement of a caloric deficit through exercise.
   b. endurance activity is most helpful in increasing caloric expenditure.
   c. resistance activity, which is low in caloric cost, acts directly to maintain or even increase muscle mass
   d. a, b, and c are correct
   e. b and c are correct

Answer- b

8 The inclusion of an exercise component in a weight/fat control program:
   a. does not maintain muscle mass.
   b. allows weight to be lost at a faster rate than just dieting even if the negative caloric deficit is equal.
   c. greatly assists in the ability to maintain a weight loss.
   d. allows more empty, junk food calories to be enjoyed without affecting the weight loss and so improves psychological and physical health.

Answer- c

9. Which of the following statements is NOT true regarding the maintenance of a weight/fat loss?
   a. Lipoprotein lipase, an enzyme responsible for fat synthesis and storage, is increased in obese individuals who have lost approximately 15% of total body weight.
   b. Lipoprotein lipase activity changes are minimal after weight loss in mildly or moderately overweight individuals.
   c. Food efficiency decreases after a weight loss such that an individual needs fewer calories to sustain a given weight.
   d. Increased food efficiency operates at the two extremes of obesity and excessive thinness when the body reacts to protect against what is perceived as a wasting away.

Answer- c

10. The recommended caloric deficit and resultant weight loss are:
    a. 1000 kcal·d^{-1} for a 1 to 2 lbs per week loss.
    b. 1500 kcal·d^{-1} for a 3 lb. per week loss.
    c. 250-500 kcal·d^{-1} for a 1/2 to 1 lb. per week loss.
    d. 100 kcal·d^{-1} for a 1/4 of a lb. per week loss.

Answer- c

11. Which combination of exercises (alternated, of course) would constitute the best program for body weight/composition control assuming it is used in conjunction with a nutritionally sound but calorically restricted diet to achieve a calorie deficit?
    a. 3 days water aerobics, 3 days step aerobics, 1 day rest.
    b. 3 days step aerobics, 3 days resistance exercises, 1 day rest.
    c. 2 days lap swimming, 2 days bicycle ergometer, 2 days calisthenics, 1 day rest.
    d. 3 days running, 3 days cycling, 1 day tennis.

Answer- b

12. Spot reduction by exercising a specific anatomical location:
    a. can increase muscle tone, which may give a slimming appearance, or increase muscle hypertrophy which gives a more defined appearance, but fat is not preferentially lost at that site.
    b. is based on the fact that local chemical changes in phosphates, CO_2 and lactate stimulate local adipose sites to mobilize the fat before other stores are used.
    c. is effective in selectively removing fat stores.
    d. a, b, and c are correct
    e. b and c are correct

Answer- a

13. When using aerobic endurance activity to create a caloric deficit for weight loss, it is important to:
    a. remember that the only way to lose fat is to burn it as a fuel.
    b. find a combination that allows the individual to burn a large number of calories (200-300 kcal) even if it means de-emphasizing intensity in favor of an increased duration.
    c. use the net, not the gross caloric value in calculating caloric expenditure since the resting component would have been utilized any way.
    d. a, b, and c are correct
    e. b and c are correct

Answer- e

B. Fill in the Blank

1. Energy can neither be created nor destroyed but only changed in form is called the _____ _____.

   Answer- First Law of Thermodynamics or the Law of Conservation of Energy

2. _____ is the amount of heat needed to raise the temperature of 1 kg of water 1°C.
   Answer- Kilocalorie

3. _____ is the mathematical summation of the caloric intake (+) and energy expenditure (-) from all sources.
   Answer- Caloric Balance Equation

4. _____ is (a) The food regularly consumed during the course of normal living; (b) a restriction of caloric intake.
   Answer- Diet

5. The level of energy required to sustain the body's vital functions in the waking state, when the individual is in a fasted condition, at normal body and room temperature, and without psychological stress is called _____ _____.
   Answer- Basal Metabolic Rate (BMR)

6. The energy expended while an individual is resting quietly in a supine position is called _____ _____.

   Answer- Resting Metabolic Rate (RMR)

7. _____ are repeated bouts of weight loss and regain.
   Answer- Weight Cycling

8. _____ is the production of heat.
   Answer- Thermogenesis

9. The increased heat production as a result of food ingestion is called _____.
Answer- Thermic Effect of a Meal (TEM)

10. An index of the amount of calories an individual needs to ingest in order to maintain a given weight or percent body fat _____.
Answer- Food Efficiency

Chapter 16

SKELETAL SYSTEM
Outline

I. Introduction

II. Skeletal Tissue

    A. Functions

    B. Levels of Organization

        1. Bones as Organs

        2. Bone Tissue

    C. Bone Development

        1. Growth

        2. Modeling

        3. Remodeling

            a. Bone Cells

            b. Hormonal Control

III. Assessment of Bone Health

    A. Laboratory Measures

        1. Absorptiometry

        2. Biochemical Markers

    B. Field Tests

IV. Factors Influencing Bone Health

    A. Age-related Changes in Bone

    B. Sex Differences in Bone Mineral Density

       C.   Development of Peak Bone Mass

V.   Exercise Response

VI.   Application of the Training Principles

       A.   Specificity

       B.   Overload

       C.   Individualization

       D.   Retrogression/Plateau

       E.   Warm-up/Cool-down

VII. Skeletal Adaptations to Exercise Training

VII. Special Applications to Health and Fitness

       A.   Osteoporosis

       B.   Physical Activity, Altered Menstrual Function, and Bone Density

       C.   Skeletal Injuries

Chapter 16

SKELETAL SYSTEM
Suggested Laboratory Activities

1. If equipment is available, measure bone mineral density in as many students as possible.

2. Prepare a list of exercise modalities and /or specific workout. Have students evaluate the theoretical effectiveness of each for improving or maintaining skeletal health.

Chapter 16

SKELETAL SYSTEM
Review Questions

1. Compare and contrast cortical and trabecular bone.

   Table 16.1; Pgs. 403-404
   Both types of bone tissue contain bone cells (osteoblasts, osteoclasts, and osterocytes), organic material, and inorganic salts (hydroxyapatites) in their matrix. However, they differ in the degree to which they are calcified; cortical bone is 80-90% calcified, whereas trabecular bone is only 15-25% calcified by volume. Thus, cortical bone is better suited for the function of support and protection and trabecular bone is better suited to the metabolic functions of bone. Cortical bone is found primarily in the shafts of long and short bones and on the outside of flat and irregular bones. Trabecular bone is found to a greater extent in the epiphysis of long bones. The table below summarizes the important differences between cortical and trabecular bone.

	Cortical	Trabecular
location	shaft of long & short bones; outside of irregular bones	epiphysis of long bones; center of flat & irregular bones
function	support & protection	metabolic functions (remodeling)
% calcified	80-90%	15-25%
resistance to fractures	high	low

2. Diagram the stages of bone remodeling, citing the specific role of the bone cells.

   Figure 16.2; Pgs. 405-407
   Stage I: Bone surface is quiet. Osteoclasts are signaled to move to area (unknown reason for this response) and begin resorption. Osteoclasts move into remodeling site (bone surface) and begin resorption of bone.
   Stage II: Osteoclast activity is stopped, and osteoblasts are signaled to move to hollowed out area on bone surface and begin to deposit bone matrix. Osteoblasts move into resorbed area and deposit bone matrix.

Stage III: Osteoblasts fill resorbed cavity to some predetermined level (unknown mechanism of control).

Stage IV: Osteoblasts stop depositing bone matrix.

3. What is the relationship between hormonal control of blood calcium levels and the hormonal control of bone remodeling?

   Pgs. 406-407
   Because the body maintains the blood calcium level very closely, any changes in blood calcium level will influence the calcium levels in bone. If the blood calcium levels are low, reserves from bone tissue will be used. Conversely, if there is too much calcium in the blood, calcium deposits will be made to bone. The primary hormones involved in regulating blood calcium levels (and thus, bone remodeling) are parathyroid hormone (PTH), calcitonin, and vitamin D. Excess calcium in the blood causes the release of calcitonin which leads to deposition of calcium in the bone. Conversely, when blood calcium levels drop below normal values, PTH stimulates osteoclast activity and blood calcium levels are increased.

4. Why are osteoporotic fractures more likely to occur in bones with a higher percentage of trabecular bone than cortical bone?

   Pg. 404
   Trabecular bone is less dense and less fracture resistant than cortical bone. Furthermore, trabecular bone has a larger surface area, and is more metabolically active than cortical bone. Due to this, metabolic activity trabecular bone also has the greatest age-related bone loss. Therefore, the most common sites of osteoporotic fractures occur in the areas with a higher percentage of trabecular bone, i.e., wrist, hip and spine.

5. Why are women more likely to suffer osteoporotic fractures than men?

   Figure 16.5; Pgs. 410-411
   There is a systematic difference in the BMD between men and women. The peak BMD achieved by women is less than that of men. Also, at the time of menopause, females lose the protective influence of estrogen, and the rate of bone loss is accelerated. Thus, the difference in BMD is extenuated in the elderly.

6. What can be done during the adult years to optimize the attainment of peak bone mass? Why is the attainment of peak bone mass important?

   Pgs. 411-412
   Three factors must be addressed to optimize peak BMD; namely nutritional, hormonal, and physical activity. Mechanical factors are necessary to stimulate bone formation. This suggests that high impact weight bearing activity will have the greatest positive effect on the development of peak bone mass. Adequate nutrition (primarily calcium intake) is necessary for bone health. Also, a normal hormonal environment, especially in females, is necessary for optimal bone health. The last factor that effects bone health is genetics. Obviously, this factor cannot be changed. Attainment of optimal peak bone mass is necessary so that as a person enters the phase of normal age-related bone loss, adequate BMD will remain to protect against fracture.

7. What factors influence skeletal adaptations to exercise?

   Table 16.4; Pgs. 414-415
   Skeletal adaptation is influenced by the <u>specific</u> type of exercise training that is used and the degree to which the skeletal system is <u>overloaded</u>. Skeletal adaptation is also <u>individualized</u>, suggesting that the same exercise program will not result in the exact same skeletal adaptation in all individuals. The specificity principle, as applied to skeletal adaptation, suggests that adaptation is specific to the bones being stressed, the composition of the bone being stressed and the type of activity performed. Weight-bearing exercise leads to greater skeletal adaptation. The overload that bone is exposed to refers to the impact load. Impact loading, or exercise with high ground reaction forces, appears to lead to the greatest skeletal adaptations.

8. Why should an amenorrheic athlete seek medical advice?

   Pgs. 416-418
   Amenorrhea is associated with low estrogen levels. Low estrogen levels, among other things, is associated with decreased BMD. This makes the athletes more susceptible to stress fractures, interferes with the attainment of peak bone mass, and increases the likelihood of osteoporitic fractures later in life.

9. Describe the role of physical activity in the prevention of osteoporosis.

   Pgs. 415-418
   The exact role of physical activity in the prevention of osteoporosis is not known. It is known, however, that lack of physical activity is linked with low BMD. It is also thought that there is a threshold level of exercise that must be met to cause osteoblast activity. Physical activity should be weight-bearing in nature, high intensity, and short in duration to have the greatest positive effect on bone.

10. Defend or refute the following statements:

    Pgs. 418-419
    a) *Disturbances in bone growth frequently result from overtraining in young athletes.*

    Refute- Disturbances in bone growth do not occur directly from overtraining. A result of overtraining maybe secondary amenorrhea, which will directly influence bone health. But there is no proof that overtraining causes bone growth disturbances.

    b) *Young athletes are more susceptible to stress fractures during the time of peak growth than at other times.*

    Support- There is a growing body of evidence that the incidence of stress fractures is growing as more children and adolescents participate in competitive sports. The time of peak incidence for stress fractures can be pinpointed as between the ages of 10 and 15, at the time of peak growth. It is at this time when there is an imbalance between bone matrix formation and mineralization. This situation increases the chances of stress fractures.

Chapter 16

SKELETAL SYSTEM
Exam Questions

A. Multiple Choice

1. The process of bone remodeling serves which function?
    a. the repair of microfractures by replacing old bone tissue
    b. regulating blood Ca^{++} levels
    c. changing the shape of bones as growth occurs
    d. a and b are correct
    e. a, b, and c are correct

Answer- d

2. Which of the following are structural functions of the skeletal system?
    1. Ca^{++} and phosphate reservoir 2. White blood cell formation 3. Support
    4. Hematopoiesis 5. Protection of vital organs 6. Locomotion
    a. 1, 3, 6
    b. 3, 4, 5
    c. 3, 5, 6
    d. 1-6 are correct

Answer- c

3. Which of the following are metabolic functions of the skeletal system?
    1. Ca^{++} and phosphate reservoir 2. White blood cell formation 3. Support
    4. Hematopoiesis 5. Protection of vital organs 6. Locomotion
    a. 1, 2, 4
    b. 1, 4, 5
    c. 4, 5, 6
    d. 1-6 are correct

Answer- a

4. Osteoblasts:
    a. are mature bone cells that regulate metabolic process of bone.
    b. are resorption of bone tissue.
    c. are composed of calcium and phosphate salts.
    d. are deposition of bone tissue.

Answer- d

5. Osteoclasts:
    a. are mature bone cells that regulate metabolic process of bone.
    b. are resorption of bone tissue.
    c. are composed of calcium and phosphate salts.
    d. are deposition of bone tissue.

Answer- b

6. Osteocytes:
    a. are mature bone cells that regulates metabolic process of bone
    b. are resorption of bone tissue
    c. are composed of calcium and phosphate salts
    d. are deposition of bone tissue

Answer- a

7. Trabecular bone:
    a. has a larger surface area than cortical bone
    b. has approximately 15-25% of it's volume calcified
    c. carries out a majority of the bone's metabolic functions
    d. all of the above are correct

Answer- d

8. Place the following phases of bone remodeling in the proper sequence:
    1. Osteoblast appear 2. Osteoclast stimulated 3. Osteoid calcifies
    4. Bone matrix deposited 5. Resorption occurs
    a. 1, 5, 2, 4, 3
    b. 5, 2, 1, 4, 3
    c. 2, 5, 1, 4, 3
    d. 5, 1, 2, 4, 3

Answer- c

9. Hormones that play a primary role in the regulation of blood Ca^{++} levels and bone remodeling are:
    a. estrogen, PTH, insulin
    b. PTH, calcitonin, Vit D
    c. calcitrol, estrogen, calcitonin, thyroid hormone
    d. all sex hormones, Vit D

Answer- b

10. Your 50 year old mother, who has just had a DXA measurement of her spine and hip, has been told she is osteopenic. As an exercise leader what type of exercise do you recommend?
    a. swimming
    b. roller blading
    c. running
    d. walking

Answer- d

B. Fill in the Blank

1. The continual process of bone breakdown (resorption) and formation (deposition of new bone) is called _____ _____.
   Answer- Bone Remodeling

2. _____ _____ is the process of altering the shape of bone by bone resorption and bone deposition.
   Answer- Bone Modeling

3. _____ are bone cells that cause the resorption of bone tissue (bone-destroying cells).
   Answer- Osteoclasts

4. _____ are bone cells that cause the deposition of bone tissue (bone-forming cells).
   Answer- Osteoblasts

5. _____ are mature osteoblasts surrounded by calcified bone that help regulate the process of bone remodeling.
   Answer- Osteocytes

6. Calcium and phosphate salts that are responsible for the hardness of the bone matrix are called _____.
   Answer- Hydroxyapatite

7. A condition of decreased bone mineral density (BMD), diagnosed when BMD is greater than one standard deviation (SD) below (but not more than 2.5 SD below) values for young, normal adults is called _____.
   Answer- Osteopenia

8. _____ is a condition of porosity and decreased bone mineral density that is defined as a BMD greater than 2.5 standard deviations (SD) below values for young, normal adults.
   Answer- Osteoporosis

9. _____ _____ is a movement performed in which the body weight is supported by muscles and bones.
Answer- Weight-Bearing Exercise

10. _____ _____ is a movement performed in which the body weight is supported or suspended and thereby not working against the pull of gravity.
Answer- Non-Weight-Bearing Exercise

11. The absence of menses is called _____.
Answer- Amenorrhea

12. Maladaptive areas of bone hyperactivity where the balance between resorption and deposition is progressively lost such that resorption exceeds deposition is called _____ _____.
Answer- Stress Reactions

13. _____ _____ is a fine hairline break in bone that occurs in the absence of acute trauma, is clinically symptomatic, and is detectable by X-rays or bone scans.
Answer- Stress Fracture

Chapter 17

SKELETAL MUSCLE TISSUE
Outline

I. Introduction

II. Overview of Muscle Tissue

    A. Functions of Skeletal Muscle

    B. Characteristics of Muscle Tissue

III. Macroscopic Structure of Skeletal Muscles

    A. Organization and Connective Tissue

    B. Architectural Organization

IV. Microscopic Structure of a Muscle Fiber

    A. Muscle Fibers

        1. Sarcoplasmic Reticulum and Transverse Tubules

        2. Myofibrils and Myofilaments

        3. Sarcomeres

V. Molecular Structure of the Myofilaments

    A. Thick Filaments

    B. Thin Filaments

VI. Contraction of a Muscle Fiber

    A. The Sliding Filament Theory of Muscle Contraction

    B. Excitation-Contraction Coupling

    C. Changes in the Sarcomere During Contraction

    D. All-or-none Principle

VII. Muscle Fiber Types
   A. Assessment of Muscle Fiber Type
   B. Distribution of Fiber Types
   C. Fiber Type in Athletes

Chapter 17

SKELETAL MUSCLE TISSUE
Suggested Laboratory Activities

1. Prepare a list of sports and specific positions within a sport. Have students determine whether a predominance of fast twitch glycolytic (FG), fast twitch oxidative glycolytic (FOG), or slow twitch oxidative (SO) or a balance of fiber types would offer the best composition for success in each.

Chapter 17

SKELETAL MUSCLE SYSTEM
Review Questions

1. List, in order of largest to smallest, the major components of the whole muscle.

   Figure 17.2; Pg. 425
   Whole muscle, fasciculi, fibers, myofibrils, myofilaments
   The muscle is composed of bundles of fasciculi (wrapped by perimysium). In turn, the fasciculi is composed of many individual muscle fiber (wrapped by endomysium). The muscle fiber is composed of myofibrils which are made up of myofilaments.

2. What causes the striated appearance of skeletal muscle fibers?

   Figure 17.4; Pgs. 427
   At the microscopic level, the sarcomere contains two types of myofilaments; myosin (thick) and actin (thin). The repeating pattern of these myofilaments gives the appearance of light and dark bands, which gives skeletal muscle the striated look.

3. What are the T-tubules and the sarcoplasmic reticulum? What is the function of each?

   Figure 17.4; Table 17.1
   The T-tubules are invaginations from the cell membrane into the cell that allows the excitation (Action Potential) from the cell membrane (sarcolemma) to be spread into the interior of the cell. As the excitation travels along the T-tubules it causes the release of calcium from the sarcoplasmic reticulum. The sarcoplasmic reticulum is a network of tubules that stores calcium, and releases calcium to the myofilaments when an action potential travels along the T-tubules.

4. Relate each region of the sarcomere to the presence of thick and thin myofilaments.

   Figures 17.4-17.5; Pgs. 428-429
   The A band is composed of thick and thin filaments. Within the A band the area that contains only thick filaments is called the H zone. The I band is composed of thin filaments only.

5. Diagram a sarcomere at rest and at the end of a contraction, and identify each of the areas.

   Figure 17.12; Pg. 436

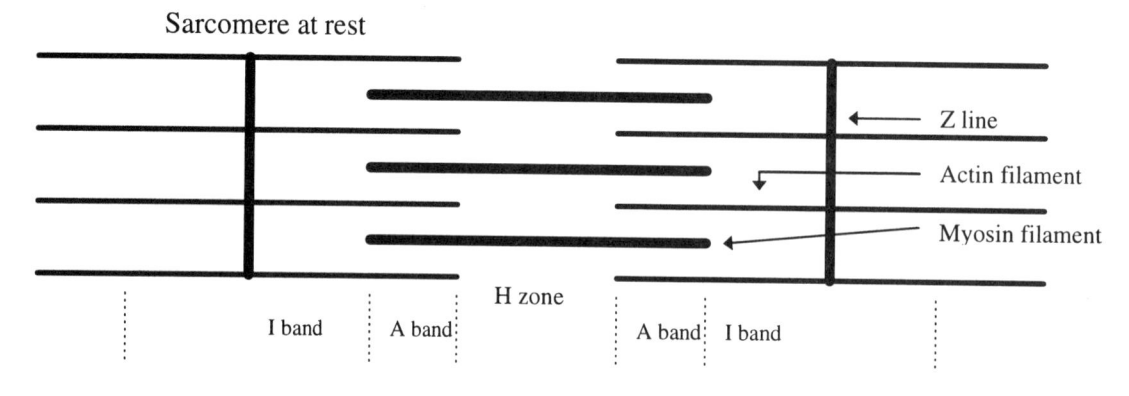

   Sarcomere at rest

   Sarcomere during contraction

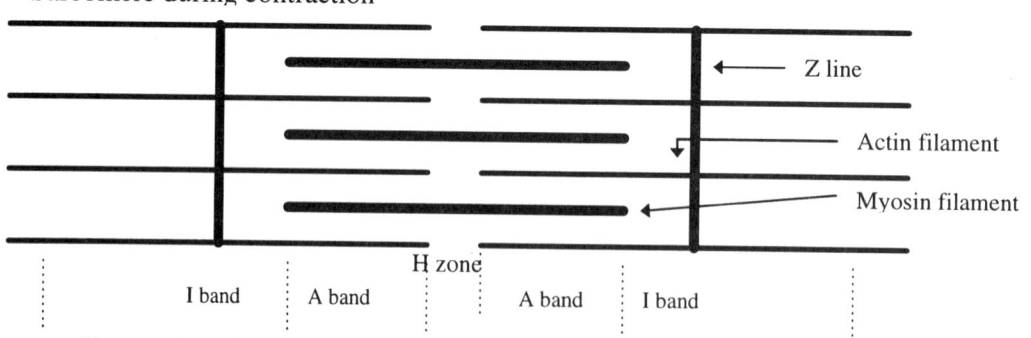

   Contraction does not change the length of the A band. This is because the length of the filaments are not compressed during contraction, rather the thin filament slides over the thick filament. As a result of the thin filament sliding over the thick filament, the H zone decreases or disappears during contraction. The sliding of the thin filaments results in a shortening of the I band and the sarcomere.

6. Describe the role of the regulatory proteins in controlling muscle contraction.

   Figure 17.9; Pg. 431
   Tropomyosin and troponin are regulating proteins found on the thin filaments which regulate the ability of myosin heads to bind to actin. Tropomyosin is a long, double stranded protein that is wrapped around the long axis of actin and blocks the active site on actin under resting conditions. Troponin is a small globular protein that controls the position of tropomyosin.
   During contraction, calcium is released from the sarcoplasmic reticulum. This calcium binds to troponin, causing it to undergo a configurational change, which causes tropomyosin to be removed from its blocking position. The myosin heads can then bind to the active sites on actin.

7. Describe the sequence of events in excitation-contraction coupling.

   Figure 17.10; Pg. 436
   Excitation-contraction coupling refers to the series of events whereby the electrical excitation in the sarcolemma of a muscle fiber leads to contraction of the muscle fiber.
   Step 1- Excitation (action potential)
   Step 2- Action potential carried to interior of the cell through the T-tubules.
   Step 3- Calcium is released from the sarcoplasmic reticulum.
   Step 4- Calcium binds to troponin, causing exposure of active site.
   Step 5- Cross-bridging cycle: Myosin heads bind to actin and swivel, pulling actin over myosin.
   Step 6- Calcium returned to sarcoplasmic reticulum; contraction ends; tropomyosin restored to blocking position.

8. Identify the role of ATP in the production of force within the contractile unit of muscle.

   Figure 17.11; Pgs. 433-436
   ATP is important for two steps in the cross bridge cycle. In order for the actin and myosin to detach, ATP must bind to myosin (step 3). The ATP that is bound to myosin is then broken down (hydrolysis) to provide the energy to activate the myosin head (step 4). This is necessary so that the myosin head can swivel during the power stroke (step 2).

9. What is the role of calcium in muscle contraction?

> **Pgs. 432-433**
> Calcium plays a key role in muscle contractions. When calcium is released from the sarcoplasmic reticulum, it binds to troponin causing tropomyosin to be removed from it's blocking position on actin. Once the active sites on actin are exposed, actin and myosin bind, leading to contraction.

10. Describe the all-or-none principle as it relates to the contraction of a single muscle fiber.

> **Pgs. 436-437**
> When a motor unit is stimulated, all the muscle fibers in the motor unit contract to their fullest extent or they do not contract al all. A muscle fiber either contracts or it does not. No partial contraction is possible.

11. Diagram the force production, twitch speed, and fatigue curve for the different fiber types.

> **Figure 17.15; Pg. 440**
> Fast glycolytic (FG) fibers produce the greatest force, but fatigue quickly.
> Slow glycolytic (SO) fibers produce the least force, but are fatigue resistant.
> Fast oxidative glycolytic (FOG) fibers are intermediate between FG and SO fibers in terms of force production and fatigue.

12. Discuss the possibility of influencing fiber type distribution by exercise training.

> **Pg. 442**
> The distribution of fiber types is based on contractile properties (slow twitch or fast twitch), is genetically determined, and does not appear to be influenced by exercise training. However, training can influence the metabolic properties of a cell. Perhaps metabolic properties can be sufficiently altered to cause a conversion of the FT fiber subdivision (e.g. FG becomes FOG).

Chapter 17

SKELETAL MUSCLE SYSTEM
Exam Questions

A. Multiple Choice

1. The four characteristics of muscle fibers which allow for movement include:
   a. irritability, excitability, conductivity and contractility
   b. irritability, contractility, extensibility and elasticity
   c. excitability, conductivity, contractility and extensibility
   d. conductivity, contractility, extensibility and irritability

Answer- b

2. Organize the following muscular tissues from most external (visible to the naked eye or simple microscope) to most internal (requires an electron microscope to view).
   1. contractile proteins
   2. endomysium
   3. epimysium
   4. fascia
   5. fasciculi
   6. muscle fiber
   7. myofibril
   8. (myo)filament
   9. perimysium

   a. 4, 2, 6, 3, 5, 8, 7, 9, 1
   b. 3, 4, 5, 2, 8, 7, 6, 1, 9
   c. 4, 3, 9, 5, 2, 6, 7, 8, 1
   d. 6, 4, 3, 5, 2, 9, 1, 7, 8

Answer- c

3. Sarcomeres:
   a. are the functional unit of the muscle fiber.
   b. extend from one z disc to the next.
   c. appear as alternating bands of light and dark striations which result from the refraction of light through the myofilaments making up the bands.
   d. a, b, and c are correct.

Answer- d

4. Within the sarcomere:
   a. the I bands contain mostly thin filaments, but overlap slightly with thick filaments.
   b. the thick filaments run the entire length of the A band.
   c. the A band is interrupted in the mid-section by the H zone where there is no overlap of thick and thin filaments.
   d. a, b, and c are correct.
   e. b and c are correct.

Answer- e

5. The filaments are comprised of contractile proteins, each of which has a characteristic appearance. Which of the following is/are accurate description(s)?
   a. Actin appears as a coiled coil. It contains active sites and is pulled toward the center of the sarcomere, during contraction.
   b. Tropomyosin (3 globular subunits) and troponin (a coiled, coiled coil) block the active site on the actin.
   c. Myosin is composed of a tail and two heads, one of which binds to ATP and the other to actin.
   d. a, b, and c are correct.
   e. a and c are correct.

Answer- e

6. Organize the following actions to accurately represent the steps in a muscle contraction for a skilled activity.
   1. Troponin undergoes conformation change
   2. Impulse travels along T-Tubules
   3. Power stroke/sliding
   4. Cross-bridging
   5. Neural impulse (action potential) originates in motor cortex
   6. Neural impulse synapses at myoneural junction
   7. Ca++ is released from Sarcoplasmic Reticulum
   8. Tropomyosin rolls deeper into groove exposing active sites
   a. 5, 2, 6, 7, 8, 1, 3, 4
   b. 6, 5, 7, 2, 1, 8, 3, 4
   c. 4, 5, 2, 6, 7, 4, 3, 8
   d. 5, 6, 2, 7, 1, 8, 4, 3

Answer- d

7. The role of ATP in skeletal muscle contraction is to:
   a. activate or energize the myosin cross bridges - this involves hydrolysis of the ATP. The enzyme myosin ATPase (myofibril ATPase) is required for this reaction.
   b. cause detachment of the myosin cross-bridges by binding to myosin after the power stroke.
   c. provide the energy for the release of calcium from its storage sacs and the return of calcium to those storage sacs.
   d. a, b, and c are correct.
   e. a and b are correct.

Answer- e

8. Cycling of the myosin cross-bridges:
   a. occurs only once for a complete shortening of the sarcomere or twitch of a muscle fiber.
   b. continues as long as calcium is bound to troponin.
   c. does not take place during eccentric contraction.
   d. a, b, and c are correct.
   e. a and b are correct.

Answer- b

9. The probable explanation for the difference in energy cost between positive and negative work is:
   a. myoglobin takes on oxygen during lengthening but must release it during shortening.
   b. lengthening involves less cycling of the cross-bridges and hence less energy.
   c. cross-bridges must be formed (thus using energy) only during shortening; lengthening is a passive process requiring no cross-bridges and thus energy only to stop the movement.
   d. fewer muscle fibers are recruited during concentric contraction than eccentric, but each works harder and burns more oxygen.

Answer- b

10. Which of the following statements is not true?
    a. Both ST and FT fiber types can create lactic acid.
    b. Males normally possess a greater percentage of Type I fibers than females.
    c. It appears that FOG fibers can be converted to FG fibers (or vice versa) through training.
    d. Both ST and FT fiber types hypertrophy with training.

Answer- b

11. Which of the following is not a true statement regarding muscle fibers and contraction?
    a. Fast twitch fibers are used preferentially for sprint-like activities whereas slow twitch fibers are used preferentially for endurance activities.
    b. There are basically two kinds of motor units: one containing fast twitch fibers and the other containing slow twitch fibers.
    c. At birth most muscle fibers are undifferentiated (Type IIc) and may be influenced by early fast or slow movements to develop into fast twitch or slow twitch fibers.
    d. For any given velocity of movement, the peak force and peak power produced are greater the higher the percentage distribution of fast twitch fibers in the muscle.

Answer- c

B. Fill in the Blank

1. The ability of a muscle to receive and respond to stimuli is called _____.
   Answer- Irritability

2. The ability of a muscle to respond to a stimuli by shortening is called _____.
   Answer- Contractility

3. The ability of a muscle to be stretched or lengthened is called _____.
   Answer- Extensibility

4. The ability of a muscle to return to resting length after being stretched is called _____.
   Answer- Elasticity

5. The _____ _____ is the specialized muscle cell organelle that stores calcium.
   Answer- Sarcoplasmic Reticulum (SR)

6. _____ _____ are organelles that carry the electrical signal form the sarcolemma into the interior of the cell.
   Answer- Transverse tubules (T tubules)

7. _____ are contractile structures composed of myofilaments.
   Answer- Myofibrils

8. Contractile (thick and thin) proteins that are responsible for muscle contraction are called _____.
   Answer- Myofilaments

9. The functional units (contractile units) of muscle fibers are called _____.
   Answer- Sarcomere

10. The _____ _____ _____ _____ _____ is the theory that explains muscle contraction as the result of the myofilaments sliding over one another.
    Answer- Sliding Filament Theory of Muscle Contraction

11. _____ _____ is the sequence of events by which an action potential in the sarcolemma initiates the sliding of the myofilaments, resulting in contraction.
    Answer- Excitation-Contraction Coupling

12. The cyclic events that are necessary for the generation of force or tension within the myosin heads during muscle contraction is called the _____ _____.
    Answer- Cross-Bridging Cycle

13. When a motor neuron is stimulated, all of the muscle fibers in that motor unit contract to their fullest extent or they do not contract at all. This is because of the _____ _____.
    Answer- All-or-None Principle

14. _____ _____ are slow-twitch muscle fibers that rely primarily on oxidative metabolism to produce energy.
    Answer- Slow Oxidative (SO) Fibers

15. _____ _____ are fast-twitch muscle fibers that have the ability to work under oxidative and glycolytic conditions.
    Answer- Fast Oxidative Glycolytic (FOG) Fibers

16. Fast-twitch muscle fibers that perform primarily under glycolytic conditions are called _____ _____.
    Answer- Fast Glycolytic (FG) Fibers

17. A motor neuron and the muscle fibers it innervates is called a _____ _____.
    Answer- Motor Unit

Chapter 18

MUSCULAR CONTRACTION AND HUMAN MOVEMENT
Outline

I. Exercise - The Result of Muscle Contraction
    A. Tension versus Load
    B. Classification of Muscle Contractions
    C. Force Development or Variation and Gradation of Response
        1. Neural Activation
        2. Mechanical Factors Influencing Muscle Contractions
            a. Length-Tension-Angle Relationships
            b. Force-Velocity and Power-Velocity Relationships
            c. Elasticity-Force Relationship
            d. Architectural Design
    D. Muscular Fatigue and Soreness
        1. Muscular Fatigue
        2. Muscular Soreness
            a. Etiology and Mechanisms
            b. Treatment for Relief and Prevention

II. Assessing Muscular Function
    A. Laboratory Methods
        1. Electromyography
        2. Isokinetic Machines
        3. Force Transducers
    B. Laboratory and Field Methods

        1. Dynamometers

        2. Constant Resistance Equipment

    C. Field Tests

        1. Calisthenic Activities

        2. Vertical Jump/Standing Broad Jump

III. Age, Sex and Muscle Function

IV. Heritability of Muscular Function

Chapter 18

MUSCULAR CONTRACTION AND HUMAN MOVEMENT
Suggested Laboratory Activities

1. Using cable tensiometers or strain gauge apparatus, determine the force (N) exerted at regular intervals between 60 degrees and 180 degrees for hip adduction and elbow extension or any other selected joint movements. Plot the resultant data to obtain strength curves. Compare and contrast the obtained strength curves with those available in the chapter.

2. Using isokinetic equipment, determine the peak torque obtained during contractions over the range of motion at a minimum of four selected speeds for one or more muscle groups. Graph the results. Dicuss the relationship between force production and velocity of shortening.

3. Have each student determine his/her maximal voluntary contraction (MVC) for handgrip strength. Have each individual attempt to hold 100% MVC as long as possible. Record the change in force exerted every 15 seconds until the force had dipped below 20% MVC. Graph the results.

4. To demonstrate concepts concerning delayed onset muscular soreness:
   - Compare the resultant delayed onset muscle soreness precipitated by a concentric versus eccentric series of contractions. Suggested activities include always lifting a dumbbell with the dominant hand and always lowering it with the non-dominant hand, or always stepping up on a bench with one leg and down with the other.
   - Measure strength before the concentric versus eccentric activity and at 24, 48, and 72 hours later.
   - Have half of the class do static stretching periodically during the 72 hour time period and the other half of the class not do any stretching.

5. Record electromyographic data from key muscle groups in several variations of any selected exercise (such as a push-up). Determine which variation works the most important muscle the hardest.

6. Determine the hamstring/quadriceps torque ratio for the left and the right legs. Interpret the results.

7. Compare and contrast 1-RM values for selected lifts between a male and a female of approximately the same size and training status for both upper and lower body muscle groups.

Chapter 18

MUSCULAR CONTRACTION AND HUMAN MOVEMENT
Review Questions

---

1. Define isotonic, isokinetic, and isometric contractions. Discuss how they relate to dynamic and static contractions.

   Table 18.1; Pgs. 446-448
   Isotonic - a muscle fiber contraction in which force production is unchanged when the muscle contracts, causing movement of an external load.
   Isokinetic - a muscle fiber contraction in which force production of the contraction is sufficient to overcome the external load.
   Isometric - a muscle fiber contraction in which force production of the contraction does not result in muscle fiber length change.

   Dynamic and static contractions refer to contractions in intact muscles of humans. Dynamic means that the contraction produced movement (either concentric or eccentric), whereas static means that the contraction does not produce meaningful movement.

2. Diagram the force-length relationship in a muscle fiber. Diagram a strength curve for biceps flexion, knee flexion, and knee extension. Discuss the relationship between the force-length relationship in the muscle fiber and in the whole muscle.

   Figures 18.2, 18.3, 18.5, 18.8; Pgs. 448-453

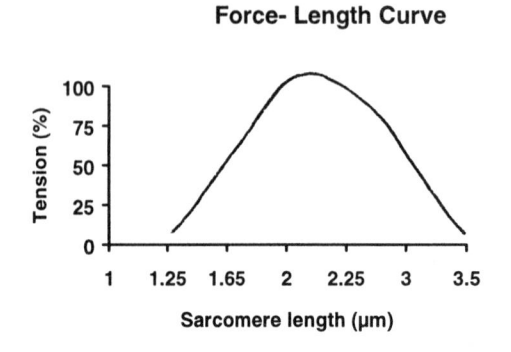

   Force- Length Curve

   (Graph: Tension (%) vs Sarcomere length (μm); curve peaks near 2–2.25 μm, with x-axis values 1, 1.25, 1.65, 2, 2.25, 3, 3.5 and y-axis values 0, 25, 50, 75, 100)

Strength Curve-biceps flexion

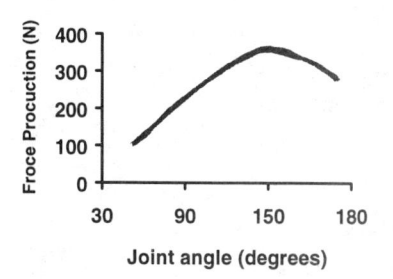

Strength Curve- knee flexion

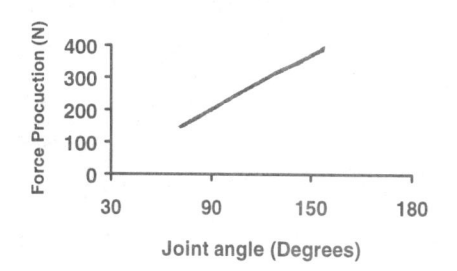

Strength Curve- knee extension

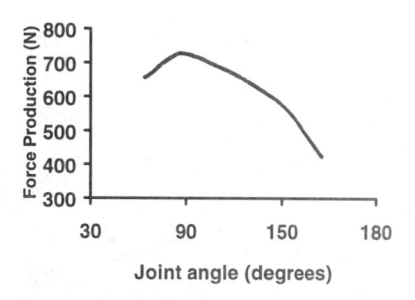

The force-length relationship is one factor that determines how much force is developed by a muscle fiber or muscle group. Within a muscle fiber, the force-length relationship can be described as essentially an inverted U-shaped relationship. The muscle fiber can exert the greatest force when the sarcomeres are at approximately 100-200% of resting length. This is because this length corresponds to the optimal amount of overlap between the thick and thin filaments.

Within the intact human muscle, the length of the muscle also affects the force that the muscle can produce. This relationship is depicted by strength curves which may be described as ascending (e.g. knee flexion), descending (e.g. hip abduction) or ascending and descending (e.g. biceps flexion and knee extension). In general, the longer the muscle length the greater the force that is exerted. It must be realized, however, that in intact human muscle, muscle length is not the only factor that determines force production The cross-sectional area of the muscle, the arrangement of the sarcomeres, the level of neural activation, the degree of fatigue, and biomechanical factors are all important.

3. Graph the force-velocity relationship in; a) a muscle fiber and b) a whole muscle. Identify the eccentric contraction on graph a and identify a static contraction on graph b.

Figures 18.10 a & b; Pgs. 453-455

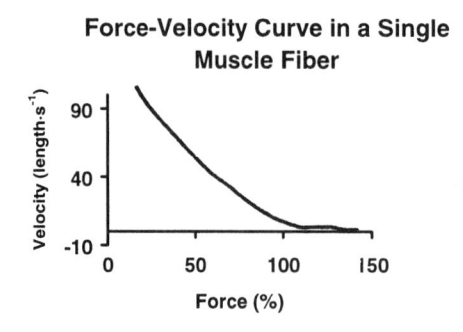

Force-Velocity Curve in a Single Muscle Fiber

Force-Velocity Curve in a Whole Muscle

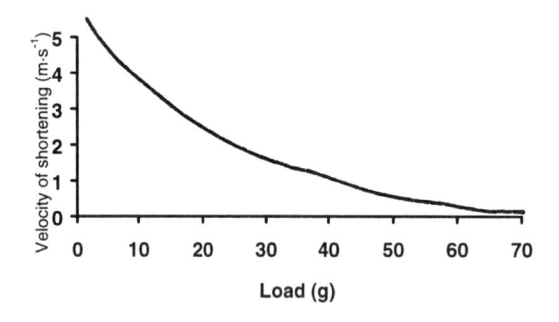

If the external force overcomes the ability of the muscle to resist it, the muscle lengthens after producing additional tension. This is an eccentric contraction.

A static contraction occurs when the load is so great that no movement (velocity or shortening) occurs.

4. Provide a schematic representation of the possible site of muscular fatigue.

Figure 18.14; Pgs. 453-455
Possible sites of fatigue can be classified central and peripheral, according to anatomical location. Central fatigue may occur anywhere in the central nervous system. Peripheral fatigue may occur in the peripheral nervous system, at the neuromuscular junction or within the skeletal muscle fibers. Additionally, the causes of fatigue may be

explained by electrophysiological considerations (within the central nervous system along the neuromuscular junction, and as the action potential is spread into the muscle fiber) or by metabolic considerations (within the muscle fiber).

5. Compare and contrast the two models proposed to explain delayed-onset muscle soreness (DOMS). Is it possible that both models are correct? Why or why not?

Figure 18.15; Pgs. 458-459
Both models propose that swelling and inflammation are what causes the sensation of pain associated with DOMS. However, the models differ in the proposed mechanisms that result in the swelling and inflammation. The mechanical trauma model suggests that high mechanical forces in the contractile elements of the muscle leads to structural damage which causes an increase in intracellular calcium, a breakdown in the regulatory proteins and an increase in immune cells (WBC). These factors then lead to inflammation and swelling.
The local ischemic model, on the other hand, suggests that overuse of muscle leads to swelling which increases tissue pressure and causes local ischemia. The local ischemia then initiates a cycle of events leading to pain, muscle spasm, more swelling and inflammation, etc. The local ischemia may also cause structural damage which would contribute to DOMS via the mechanisms described by the mechanical trauma theory.
It is likely that both theories are correct. The causative factors leading to DOMS may vary depending upon the type of exercise an individual engages in.

6. What are the primary laboratory methods of assessing muscular function? What are the primary field tests to assess muscular function? What are the limitations of the various methods? What determines which is the appropriate test to administer?

Pgs. 462-464
The primary laboratory methods of assessing muscular function are electromyography, isokinetic machines, force transducers, dynamometers, constant resistance equipment, and field tests (calisthenics, vertical and standing broad jump). Electromyography is an instrument that provides a direct functional indication of muscle activity by measuring neural or electrical activity. Isokinetic machines are instruments that allow the velocity of the limb movement to be held constant to provides accurate measurements of muscular strength, endurance and power. Force transducers are instruments that measure static strength and endurance. When an individual contracts against a force transducer, the displacement of the transducer causes an electrical signal to be sent to a computer which displays the force

output in digital form. Laboratory field methods of testing muscular function may also include dynamometers, instruments that measure static strength and endurance, usually of the handgrip or the back and leg. Constant resistance equipment is most often used to measure a person's singular maximal load measured from free weights or weight machines. The equipment can also be used to determine a person's dynamic endurance by measuring how many times an individual can lift a submaximal load. Field tests used to measure muscular function include various calisthenic activities and the vertical and/or standing broad jump.

A limitation of electromyography is that it does not give an absolute value of force or torque. Dynamometers only measure hand grip and back/leg strength. A limitation of constant resistance equipment is that maximal strength or torque is determined by trial and error, therefore a subject may be able to lift more weight than determined due to muscular fatigue resulting from several trials. It is also difficult to isolate individual muscle groups with constant resistant equipment. Calisthenics often measure endurance more than strength and are often performed poorly limiting their usefulness.

7. Compare male and female strength development during childhood and adolescence.

Pg. 464
During early childhood there is virtually no difference in strength measurement between boys and girls. As puberty begins, the gap widens between the strength measures of boys and girls. Girls between 11-12 years of age can achieve about 90 percent of a boy's strength At age 13-14, a girl achieves around 80 percent of her countersex's strength, and by the time a girl is 15-16 years, she can achieve about 75 percent of a boy's strength in her age group.

8. Discuss differences in strength between adult males and females. How is the deference in strength affected by the units used to express strength (that is, absolute or relative values)? How does it vary among different regions of the body? What is the most likely causes of sex-related differences in muscular function?

Pgs. 464-467

Strength of Females Expressed Relative to Males (%)

	Absolute	**Absolute/ Body Weight**	**Absolute/ LBM**
Handgrip	57	73	83
Bench Press	37	46	53
Leg Press	73	92	106

Differences in strength are related to the units used to express strength. On an absolute basis, women are 37-73% as strong as men for various muscle groups. However, when relative units are used (i.e., strength divided by body weight or strength divided by LBM) the difference between strength is greatly reduced or may be non-existent.

The likely reason for the difference in strength between men and women is that during puberty males produce more testosterone whereas women produce more estrogen. Testosterone aids the anabolic process of muscle growth while estrogen is involved in fat deposition in women; therefore men have a higher percentage of lean body tissue than women.

9. What factors account for the age-related decline in muscular strength? Can this loss be minimized or slowed? If so, how?

Pgs. 464-467

The factors that account for age-related muscular strength loss are loss of muscle mass, loss of mechanical or contractile properties (fiber type, size and number changes) and reduced activation of motor unites or denervation. Strength is maintained up to the age of 45-50 years. At this point, a person's strength begins to decrease at a gradual rate until approximately age 70, when the strength loss is about 30% per decade. This loss can be minimized or stopped though through a systematic exercise training program which would increase muscular strength, power, and endurance.

10. What is the role of genetics in determining an individuals' strength or an individuals' response to a training program?

   Pg. 468
   The role of genetics in determining an individuals strength or response to a training program is difficult to determine precisely due to sampling and population variation, methodical differences and a large variation of physical activity levels. However, most studies suggest that genetics determine between 20-40% of muscular strength and endurance. The expression of muscular function is determined largely by the fiber type distribution and metabolic properties of muscle fibers, both of which are influenced by genetics. Genetics account for a substantial fraction of the individual differences in determining a person response to a training program. Individuals may be a "high responder" or a "low responder" to exercise. This helps to explain why even when a number of individuals engage in a training program, different results should be expected.

Chapter 18

MUSCULAR CONTRACTION AND HUMAN MOVEMENT
Exam Questions

A. Multiple Choice

1. At approximately 110-120 percent of its resting length, a sarcomere:
   a. exerts its greatest tension because the actin filaments are pulled out of range of the cross bridges.
   b. exerts its lowest possible tension because there is an overlap of actin filaments such that the filament from one side interferes with the coupling potential of the cross bridges on the other side.
   c. exerts its greatest tension because at this length the greatest number of myosin can connect with actin filaments.
   d. can exert an amount of tension approaching zero because the actin and myosin have overlapped as much as possible.

   Answer- c

2. Match the classification of muscle contraction at the single fiber/motor unit level (first letter) with corresponding intact human classification (second letter).
   A. Dynamic   D. Isometric
   B. Isokinetic   E. Isotonic
   C. Isokinematic   F. Static
   a. E - E; B - B; D - D
   b. E - A; B - C; D - F
   c. E - A; C - B; F - F
   d. A - C; B - F; D - E

   Answer- b

3. The most likely site and cause of muscular fatigue are:
   a. the motor nerve inability to restore resting membrane potential due to leakage of K+.
   b. the neuromuscular junction due to a depletion of the neurotransmitter acetylcholine.
   c. within the contractile mechanism primarily because of metabolic factors.
   d. at the level of the central nervous system based on feedback from the contractile mechanisms.

   Answer- c

4. The most probably cause for immediate (during and right after) localized soreness of a muscle is:
   a. rupture of muscle tissue.
   b. connective tissue pull-tension.
   c. spasm initiated by ischemia.
   d. metabolites increase (i.e. lactic acid).

Answer- d

5. The most probable cause(s) for delayed (24 to 48 hrs) muscle soreness is:
   a. rupture/tear of connective tissue and muscle fiber spasm.
   b. rupture/tear of muscle fibers spasm and lactic acid.
   c. build up of PC.
   e. metabolites.

Answer- a

6. Which of the following situations is most likely to cause muscle soreness?
   a. negative workout where a spotter assists with the lifting phase but not the lowering phase.
   b. running the two mile.
   c. running the Russian lay-up drill in basketball (that is sprinting to the opposite basket after each shot).
   d. practicing back dives from the high board.

Answer- a

7. The influence of muscle fiber type on the force-velocity curve relationship shows that:
   a. the peak torque (force x lever arm or movement arm distance) generated by a muscle decreases with increasing velocities of movement regardless of the fiber type distribution.
   b. at any given velocity of movement, the torque produced is greater the lower the percentage of fast twitch fibers.
   c. at any given torque produced, the velocity of movement is greater the higher the percentage of distribution of slow twitch fiber.
   d. athletes such as downhill skiers and orienteers exhibit identical curves, which indicates that training per se does not influence the curve.

Answer-a

8. Nautilus equipment:
   a. is an example of true isokinetic contraction such that maximal tension develops in the muscle while shortening at constant speed over the full range of motion.
   b. is developed around the concept of eccentric contraction, i.e. - negative work in resisting gravity.
   c. compensates for variations in muscular force at different joint angles by changing the lever arm such that the muscle exerts near maximal force over the full range of motion.
   d. provides static resistance over a wide variety of angles.

Answer- c

9. Which of the following types of contractions develops the greatest force?
   a. eccentric dynamic
   b. concentric dynamic
   c. static
   d. isokinetic concentric

Answer- d

10. An individual was tested with the following results:
    Angle pull (E)   40   80   120 160 200
    Pounds pulled (max lb.) 40   60   90   65   60
    What is the greatest amount of weight that can be lifted (isotonically, concentrically) over the full range of motion for this individual?
    a. 40
    b. 60
    c. 65
    d. 90

Answer- a

B. Fill in the Blank

1. The capability of a force to produce rotation is called _____.
   Answer- Torque

2. A muscle fiber contraction in which the tension generated by the muscle is constant through the range of motion is called an _____ _____.
   Answer- Isotonic contraction

3. _____ _____ is a muscle contraction in which the force exerted varies as the muscle shortens to accommodate change in muscle length and/or joint angle throughout the range of motion while moving a constant external load.
   Answer- Dynamic contraction

4. _____ _____ is a dynamic muscle contraction that produces tension during shortening.
Answer- Concentric contraction

5. _____ _____ is a dynamic muscle contraction that produces tension (force) while lengthening.
Answer- Eccentric contraction

6. A muscle fiber contraction in which the velocity of the contraction is kept constant is called an _____ _____.
Answer- Isokinetic Contraction

7. A muscle contraction in which the rate of limb displacement or joint rotation is held constant with the use of specialized equipment is called an _____ _____.
Answer- Isokinematic contraction

8. A muscle fiber contraction that does not result in a length change in muscle fiber is called an _____ _____.
Answer- Isometric Contraction

9. A muscle contraction that produces an increase in muscle tension but does not cause meaningful limb displacement or joint displacement and therefore does not result in movement of the skeleton is called an _____ _____.
Answer- Static contraction

10. _____ _____ _____ is the maximal force (100%) that a muscle can exert.
Answer- Maximal Voluntary Contraction

11. _____ _____ _____ is muscle soreness that increases in intensity for the first 24 hr after activity, peaks from 24 to 28 hr, and then declines during the next 5 to 7 days.
Answer- Delayed-Onset Muscle Soreness (DOMS)

12. The ability of a muscle or muscle group to exert maximal force against a resistance in a single repetition is called _____.
Answer- Strength

13. _____ _____ is the ability of a muscle or muscle group to repeatedly exert force against a resistance.
Answer- Muscular Endurance

14. _____ is the amount of work done per unit of time; the product of force and velocity; the ability to exert force quickly.
Answer- Power

15. The measurement of the neural or electrical activity that brings about muscle contraction is called _____.
Answer- Electromyography (EMG)

Chapter 19

MUSCLE FUNCTION AND TRAINING PRINCIPLES
Outline

I. Introduction

II. Muscular Training

    A. Overview of Tesistance Training

III. Application of the Training Principles

    A. Specificity

    B. Overload

    C. Adaptation

    D. Progression

    E. Individualization

    F. Maintenance

    G. Retrogression/Plateau/Reversibility

    H. Warm-Up and Cool Down

    I. Specific Application of Training Principles to Body Building

IV. Muscular Adaptations to Exercise Training

    A. Neromuscular Adaptations to Resistance Training Programs

    B. Muscle Adaptations to Endurance Training Programs

V. Special Applications

    A. Muscular Strength and Endurance and Lower-Back Pain

    B. Anabolic Steroids

Chapter 19

MUSCULAR TRAINING PRINCIPLES AND ADAPTATIONS
Suggested Laboratory Activities

1. Measure 1-RM for a variety of dynamic resistance lifts. Count the number of repetitions that can be completed at 90% 1-RM, 80% 1-RM, 70% 1-RM, and 60% 1-RM. Graph the relationships between % 1-RM and repetitions.

2. Have students write a resistance training program for either strength, muscular endurance, power or hypertrophy and explain how each training principle is incorporated in the program.

3. Have students write a periodization cycle showing variations in training volume.

4. Prepare a variety of resistance training workouts. Have students determine the primary goal of each (strength, muscular endurance, power, or hypertrophy).

5. Compare and contrast 1-RM for selected lifts between:
    - an aerobically trained individual and a resistance trained individual (same sex)
    - a resistance trained individual and an untrained individual (same sex)

6. Determine abdominal strength/endurance and back extensor strength/endurance.

7. Compare and contrast the strength measured in any given muscle or muscle group by static, dynamic concentric, dynamic eccentric, and isokinetic techniques.

Chapter 19

MUSCULAR TRAINING PRINCIPLES AND ADAPTATIONS
Review Questions

1. Give several reasons why an individual may engage in a resistance training program, and specify the different goals of a program.

   Pg. 472
   An individual may engage in a resistance training program to improve overall health, improve athletic performance, rehabilitate an injury, change his/her physical appearance, or to compete in powerlifting or body building. A person who desires to better his/her overall health would probably train two to three times a week with a general training program to improve the muscular strength and endurance of all the major muscle groups A powerlifter would probably train 5-6 days per week with an intense training program to cause muscular hypertrophy and increased muscular strength. How one designs the training program largely depends on the extent of the results desired i.e.; muscular strength, muscular endurance, power, muscular hypertrophy or a combination of the above.

2. Discuss how each of the training principles is applied in the development of a resistance training program. How do these applications vary if the exerciser is a child?

   Pgs. 472-477
   - *Specificity*: The exerciser would design the program to achieve his/her own personal goals, be it an improvement of muscular strength and endurance or an increase in power, etc. Specificity also applies to the specific muscle groups to be exercised. This is true for an adult or a child.
   - *Overload*: As long as continued improvement is sought, overload of the muscle groups (by increasing the duration, frequency or intensity) must occur. Application of the overload principle is very similar in children but requires a few modifications. The

training program for a child should stress proper technique and safety considerations and maximal lifts should be avoided.
- *Adaptation*: When a muscle is chronically stressed, it eventually adapts to the stress placed on it. Adaptation occurs in children as it does in adults, however, careful monitoring to ensure adequate recovery periods is even more important in children than adults.
- *Progression*: Once the body has adapted to the current training level, the exercise stress must be increased according to the overload principle if further improvement is desired. Progression should be done gradually, especially in children. This is often accomplished by increasing the number of repetitions within a set, then increasing the load. Loads heavier than 6 RM are not recommended for prepubescent children.
- *Individualization*: This principle dictates that each training program be designed for an individual based on goals and an evaluation of current strength level. Furthermore, an individuals response to a training program is determined by age, body size and type, initial fitness, and genetics. Individualizing a resistance program is even more important for children than for adults.
- *Retrogression/Plateau/Reversibility*: Despite adherence to a training program there are periods when performance stays the same (plateau) or decreases (retrogression). This may indicate overtraining or it may simply be indicative of individual differences. Detraining (reversibility) occurs when an individual discontinues training. Children also detrain, although the concomitant effects of growth-related strength increases may mask it.
- *Warm-Up and Cool-Down*: A warm-up period raises body temperature and decreases the risk of injury or soreness. A cool-down period may help prevent soreness and increase flexibility. These are as important for children as adults.

3. Is there an ideal number of repetitions and sets that should be performed by everyone? If so, what is it?

   Figure 19.1; Pg. 473
   No, there is no ideal number of repetitions and sets that should be performed by all people who engage in resistance training. The ideal number of repetitions and sets are regulated by the individual goals of each person engaged in training. In general, a higher load and few reps (3-6 reps per set for 3-5 sets) is more advantageous for developing strength, whereas a lighter load and more reps are used for those seeking to develop muscular endurance.

4. Discuss the importance of adequate recovery time in training adaptations to a resistance training program.

> **Pg. 475**
> It is important for an individual to allow proper recovery time in a training program to allow for the positive adaptations of exercise training and help prevent injury and soreness. It is not beneficial to overstress the body. Therefore, it is important that at least a 24 hour rest period is granted to whatever muscle group is worked. Also, the alternation of "heavy" and "light" days is useful in the prevention of injury and soreness.

5. Do all individuals respond to a training program with the same adaptation (or magnitude of adaptation)? Why or why not?

> **Pgs. 475-476**
> No, not all individuals respond to a training program with the exact same magnitude of adaptation. This occurs because each individual has unique factors (age, body size and type, initial strength, and genetic makeup) which make him or her different from all other people, therefore, each person responds to exercise differently.

6. What is the importance of a warm-up period prior to resistance training?

> **Pg. 477**
> The importance of a proper warm-up period prior to training is that it raises the body temperature which is recommended to help prevent injury and muscle soreness. An increased body temperature decreases the viscosity of the joint capsule, increases the speed of contraction, and speeds up the enzymatic reactions

7. Compare and contrast the training adaptations that occur in skeletal muscle as a result of resistance training and endurance training.

> **Pgs. 478-481**
> Skeletal muscle responds to resistance training by increasing the strength and cross sectional area of the muscle. Slow and fast twitch muscle fibers both increase in fiber area, however, the fast twitch fibers appear to increase to a greater extent. Skeletal muscle has been recorded to increase in both men and woman who engage in a resistance training program and it occurs in all age groups. Skeletal muscle responds to endurance training by an increase in slow twitch fibers and there is some evidence that endurance training can result in the transformation of FTb fibers to FTa fibers. Endurance training in older men and women can increase the cross

sectional area of the slow twitch fibers and increase the percentage of FTa fibers. Therefore, skeletal muscle responds similarly to both types of training programs in regard to increasing slow twitch fibers. In contrast, endurance training can result in transformation of subpopulation of FT fibers whereas resistance training does not appear to do so.

8. What is the relationship between muscle function and lower-back pain.

   Pg. 481
   To maintain a healthy back, one needs to have a flexibility in the lower back muscles, hamstrings, and hip flexors. It is also important to have strong abdominal and back muscles. Research has shown that people who suffer from LBP exhibit lower levels of strength in both the abdominal and back extensors. However, this is more likely to result from LBP than to cause it.

9. Why are anabolic steroids dangerous?

   Pgs. 481-482
   Anabolic steroid use is dangerous to the body because they have adverse affects on the liver, the cardiovascular system, the male reproductive system, the female reproductive system as well as the psychological status of individuals. Anabolic steroid use has been found to have long term and short term negative effects.

Chapter 19

MUSCULAR TRAINING PRINCIPLES AND ADAPTATIONS
Exam Questions

A. Multiple Choice

1. When designing a resistance (weight) training program, it is recommended that:
   a. exercises for the lower and upper body be alternated within a given session or on different days.
   b. that small muscle groups be exercised first, followed by large muscle groups.
   c. at least one exercise be included for all major muscle groups of the body.
   d. a, b, and c are correct
   e. a and c are correct

   Answer- e

2. Which of the following exercise prescriptions should be most effective for developing muscular strength?
   a. 5 sets   12-15 RM   5 days/wk   :30 rest between sets
   b. 3 sets   6-12 RM   3 days/wk   1:30 rest between sets
   c. 3 sets   3- 6 RM   4 days/wk   3:00 rest between sets
   d. 4 sets   20-30 RM   4 days/wk   2:00 rest between sets

   Answer- c

3. Physiological adaptations to dynamic resistance training include:
   a. hypertrophy and hyperplasia of muscle fibers.
   b. improved neural activation at neuromuscular junctions and decreased inhibitory control of muscles.
   c. a toughening and thickening of connective tissue.
   d. a, b, and c are correct
   e. b and c are correct

   Answer- e

4. In order to maintain strength and endurance developed by a comprehensive dynamic resistance program, it is necessary to maintain intensity and do:
   a. 3 sets   6 RM   1 day every 1-2 wks
   b. 3 sets   10 RM at   1/2, 3/4 and RM - 1 day/every 2 wks
   c. 2 sets   10 RM   3 days/wk
   d. 3 sets   6 RM   3-4 days/wk alternately

Answer- a

5. Strength gains:
   a. do not proceed at a constant rate. They are highest initially and decrease as the program continues over a period of months.
   b. do not proceed at a constant rate. They are very slow intially when strength is a small proportion of maximal and more rapid as a greater % of maximal is reached.
   c. do not follow any consistent pattern.
   d. proceed at a constant rate.

Answer- a

6. Which of the following are typical adaptation to resistance training:
   a. increase in fiber area of ST and FT muscle fibers
   b. increase in fiber area of ST muscle fibers
   c. increase in fiber area of FT muscle fibers
   d. increase in fiber area of FOG muscle fibers

Answer- a

7. It is estimated the _____ % of all individuals experience LBP at some time in their life?
   a. < 25%
   b. 30-50%
   c. 60-80%
   d. > 90%

Answer- c

8. It has been shown that people suffering from LBP have:
   a. lower levels of strength in the abdominals and knee extension
   b. lower levels of strength in the abdominal and back extensors
   c. lower levels of strength in the back extensors and higher levels of strength in the hip flexors
   d. lower levels of strength in the back extensors and hip flexors

Answer- b

9. Anabolic steroids:
    a. are legal in some European countries.
    b. such as testosterone, will not harm females who take them.
    c. are safe if used properly under a physician's care.
    d. are synthetic androgens.

Answer- d

B. Fill in the Blank

1. _____ _____ is a systematic program of exercises involving the exertion of force against a load used to develop strength, endurance, and/or hypertrophy of the muscular system.
   Answer- Resistance Training

2. _____ is decreasing body fat and body water content to very low levels in order to increase muscle definition.
   Answer- Cutting

3. Synthetic androgens that mimic the effects of the male hormone testosterone are called _____ _____.
   Answer- Anabolic Steroids

Chapter 20

NEURAL CONTROL OF MOVEMENT
Outline

I. Introduction

II. Neural Control of Muscle Fibers

    A. Nerve Supply

    B. The Neuromuscular Junction

III. Reflex Control of Movement

    A. Spinal Cord

        1. Pyramidal System

        2. Extrapyramidal System

    B. Components of a Reflex Arc

    C. Proprioceptors and Reflexes

        1. Vestibular Apparatus

        2. Muscle Spindles and the Myotatic Reflex

        3. Golgi Tendon Organ

        4. Myotatic Reflex

IV. Volitional Control of Movement

    A. Volitional Control of Individual Motor Units

    B. Volitional Control of Muscle Movement

V. Flexibility

    A. Assessing Flexibility

    B. The Influence of Age and Sex on Flexibility

    C. Flexibility and Low-Back Pain

        D. Flexibility Training

VI.   Application of the Training Principles

        A. Specificity

        B. Overload

        C. Adaptation and Progression

        D. Individualization

        E. Maintenance

        F. Retrogression/Plateau/Reversibility

        G. Warm-Up and Cool-Down

VII.   Adaptation to Flexibility Training

Chapter 20

NEUROMUSCULAR ASPECTS OF MOVEMENT
Suggested Laboratory Activities

1. Assign various joints or muscle groups to specific class members so that as many joints or muscle groups are included as possible. Have each student design a static CR-PNF, and CRAC-PNF exercise and lead the class in at least one of these.

2. Measure lumbar, hamstring, and hip flexor range of motion with laboratory instrumentation. Perform the one legged sit-and-reach. Relate the sit-and-reach results to the laboratory measurements.

3. Compare and contrast the flexibility among athletes from different sports or individuals using different training modalities over a variety of joints.

4. Compare and contrast the flexibility among athletes from different sports or individuals using different raining modalities over a variety of joints.

5. Compare and contrast the flexibility in at least three joints between the males and the females in the class.

Chapter 20

NEUROMUSCULAR ASPECTS OF MOVEMENT
Review Questions

1. Describe the anatomical relationship between nerve and muscle. What is the functional significance of this relationship?

    Figure 20.2; Pgs. 486-487
    A motor neuron extends toward but does not actually touch skeletal muscle fibers. The area between the neuron and the muscle fiber is called the neuromuscular junction. Skeletal muscles require nervous stimulation to produce the electrical excitation in the muscle cells which leads to contraction. The significance of this relationship is that a muscle cannot move without the nervous system. If the neural connection to a muscle is damaged, it will affect the way the muscle moves or cause it's inability to move.

2. Diagram the sequence of events that occur at the neuromuscular junction.

    See Figure 20.3; Pgs. 487-489
    The sequence of events at the neuromuscular junction are as follows:
    a. an action potential (AP) is generated in the motor neuron
    b. neurotransmitter (NT) is released from the axon terminal of the motor neuron
    c. the NT diffuses across the synaptic cleft
    d. the NT binds to receptors on the sarcolemma of the muscle fiber
    e. binding of NT causes changes in membrane permeability, which initiate an AP in the muscle fiber

3. Diagram the components of a generalized reflex arc.
   See Figure 20.5; Pgs. 490-491
   A generalized reflex is composed of a receptor, an afferent neuron, an association neuron, an efferent neuron, and an effector organ.

4. Diagram the components of the myotatic reflex. Pay careful attention to the afferent and efferent neurons involved.
   See Figure 20.7; Pgs. 493-495

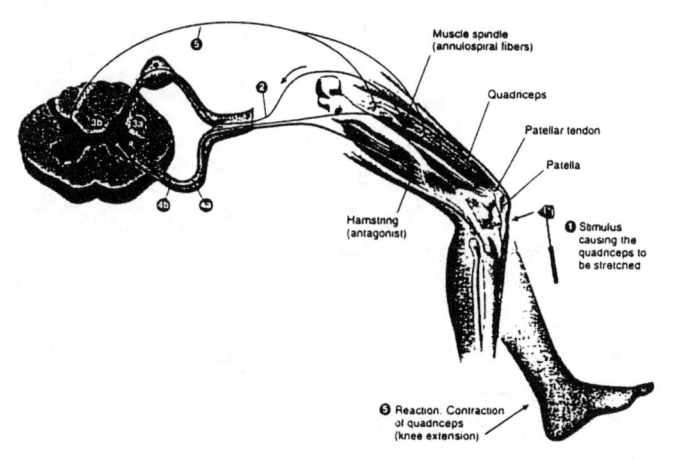

5. Diagram the components of the inverse myotatic reflex.
   See Figure 20.9; Pgs. 495-496

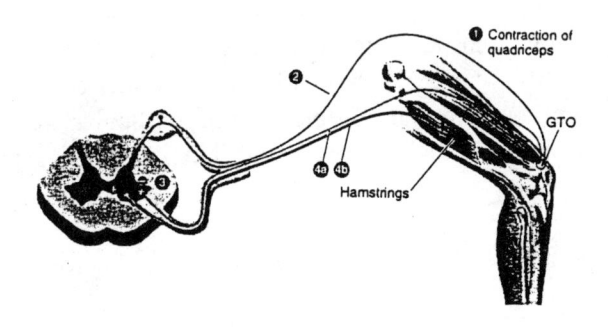

6. Outline the sequence of events involved in volitional control of movement.

See Figure 20.11; Pgs. 496-498
A. The motor cortex of the brain initiates a movement.
B. Information is transmitted down the appropriate descending pathway.
C. The information is carried to the target organ (muscle) in the periphery by an efferent motor neuron.
D. The nervous stimulation causes the muscle to contract.
E. Contraction of the muscle then stimulates the receptors located in and near the contracting muscle.
F. Information then received from the receptors is then transmitted to the spinal cord by the afferent neurons.
G. In the spinal cord:
   1. Some of the afferent neurons synapse directly with the motor neurons to cause a reflex action.
   2. Other afferent neurons synapse with neurons in the ascending pathways.
H. The brain then processes and integrates the information from the ascending pathway and other receptors.
I. The brain then transmits the information down the appropriate descending pathway.
J. B-I is repeated until the movement ends.

7. Provide a rationale for incorporating a flexibility training program into an overall fitness program.

Pgs. 498-500
Flexibility is important for daily living and for muscle relaxation and proper posture. Flexibility should be included in an overall fitness program. Stretching will prepare the muscles for a particular activity which will enhance performance and decrease the likelihood of injury during that physical activity.

8. Critique the appropriateness of the sit-and-reach test to predict low-back pain.

Pgs. 500-501
The sit and reach test is a measurement of hamstring flexibility, not lower back (lumbar) flexibility. Therefore, to use the sit and reach test to predict LBP from a measurement of hamstring flexibility and presumed low back flexibility is an incorrect use of the test.

9. What are the anatomical requirements of a healthy low back?

Pgs. 502-503
The anatomical requirements of a healthy low back are flexibility in the low back and hip region and strong, balanced lumbar, hamstrings, and hip flexor muscles for controlled pelvic movement. If one has controlled back movement, one does not have an exaggerated anterior tilt (lordotic curve) nor a restricted anterior tilt (no low back curvature). An exaggerated or restricted anterior pelvic tilt can cause an increased vertebral disc compression and cause pain and strain in the lower back.

10. Describe static stretching, and explain the involvement of reflexes in providing for muscle elongation during this type of stretching.

Pgs. 503-504
Static stretching is a form of stretching in which the muscle to be stretched is slowly put into a position of controlled maximal or near-maximal stretch. The neuromuscular system is not stimulated so reflex contraction does not occur. Instead, the GTO are stimulated, leading to the inverse myotatic reflex and thus relaxation (elongation) of the stretched muscle.

11. Describe the proprioceptive neuromuscular facilitation technique, and explain the involvement of reflexes in providing for muscle elongation during this type of stretching.

Pg. 504
Proprioceptive neuromuscular facilitation is a stretching technique in which the muscle to be stretched is first contracted maximally. The muscle is then relaxed and is either actively stretched by contraction of the opposing muscle or is passively stretched.
CR technique- The exerciser contracts the antagonists against the resistance provided by a partner. As tension is created in the muscle by the maximal contraction, the GTOs respond and the inverse myotatic reflex is initiated, resulting in a relaxation of the stretched muscle group. At this point, the partner who has been resisting the contraction moves the relaxed limb into a greater stretch.
CRAC technique- In this technique, the exerciser actively contracts the agonist to assist the stretching of the antagonist. By reciprocal inhibition, the contraction of the agonist is thought to aid in the relaxation of the antagonist, allowing it to be stretched further.

12. Discuss the application of the individual training principles to the development of a flexibility program.

   Pgs. 505-507
   - *Specificity:* Flexibility is joint specific, therefore in an exercise program one needs to analyze the task or sport and then determine the specific joints that need to be stretched.
   - *Overload:* For flexibility, overload is achieved by placing the muscle and connective tissue at or near the normal limits of extensibility and manipulating the NMS and GTO by holding the position or contracting the muscle to achieve an elongation. Duration should be 30-60 seconds, intensity should be monitored by myoclonus and pain, and frequency should be at least 3 days per week.
   - *Adaptation and progression:* Short term improvement can be seen in as little as one week. Progression will occur naturally if stretch is done to myoclonus.
   - *Individualization:* Most importantly are the goals and needs of the participant and the techniques preferred for stretching. Amount of improvement largely determined by genetics.
   - *Maintenance:* Once the desired flexibility is achieved, it can be maintained with one day of stretching per week.
   - *Retrogression and plateau:* Little is know about plateau in a flexibility training program. However, there will obviously be a point when genetics dictate no further improvement.
   - *Warm-up and cool-down:* Stretching does not increase body temperature. Therefore, it is not considered a technique of warming-up. A cardiovascular warm-up should precede the stretching so as to increase muscle and joint temperatures, decrease viscosity, and prevent muscle injury.

Chapter 20

NEUROMUSCULAR ASPECTS OF MOVEMENT
Exam Questions

A. Multiple Choice

1. The only test of muscle function which has been shown to be predictive of first time <u>and</u> recurrent episodes of low back pain is:
    a. abdominal strength/endurance: curl-ups.
    b. back extensor endurance.
    c. hamstring flexibility: back-saver sit-and-reach.
    d. lumbar flexibility: modified Schober degrees of flexion.

Answer- b

2. The physiological mechanism(s) underlying plyometrics is/are:
    a. elasticity - force relationship. When a muscle fiber is stretched and then contracted, the resultant contraction is stronger.
    b. firing of the myotatic reflex. During the eccentric phase neuromuscular spindles are activated enhancing the concentric muscle contraction.
    c. force - velocity relationship. The greater the force of the eccentric contraction phase is the greater the velocity during the concentric phase due to the optimization of the sarcomere length.
    d. a, b, and c are correct.
    e. a and b are correct.

Answer- e

3. Match the flexibility type in Column A with the proprioceptor primarily responsible in Column B.

   Column A | Column B
   A. Ballistic | D. Golgi Tendon Organ
   B. Proprioceptive Neuromuscular Facilitation (PNF) | E. Pacinian Corpuscle
   C. Static | F. Neuromuscular Spindle

    a. A - D; B - E; C - F
    b. A - E; B - F; C - D
    c. A - F; B - D; C - D
    d. A - D; B - F; C - F

Answer- c

4. An individual completes the following exercise.
   Body position: lying prone, jump rope held in both hands and wrapped around foot; knee flexed against buttocks.
   Action - rope is shortened raising knee off ground; quadriceps contract statically against taut rope 6 sec; hamstrings contract as rope is pulled tighter stretching quad. This is an example of a:
   a. Ballistic stretch
   b. PNF - CR stretch
   c. PNF - CRAC stretch
   d. Static stretch

Answer- c

5. Myoclonus:
   a. is a sign that a muscle is stretched too far and is reflexly trying to contract.
   b. is the feedback of sensory information about head position and linear acceleration via the inner ear.
   c. is responsible for the spotting technique which allows figure skaters to spin rapidly without vertigo.
   d. is the process whereby myosin and myoglobin increase during strength training.

Answer- a

6. Stretching:
   a. does not cause an elevation in body temperature and therefore cannot be considered a warm-up.
   b. should follow a cardiovascular warm-up to elevate body temperature regardless of the reason for stretching.
   c. for flexibility gains is no different after a short (3-4 min) or long (23-34 min) period of cardiovascular endurance activity.
   d. a, b, and c are correct

Answer- d

7. A normal healthy individual attempts to lift a heavy load and his muscles "give out." After this experience there is no apparent problem in neuromuscular function. What is the most likely mechanism responsible for the abrupt cessation of muscle contraction?
   a. the activation of the Golgi Tendon organs.
   b. the activation of the receptors in the annulospiral endings.
   c. skeletal muscle ischemia.
   d. the inactivation of stretch receptors in the annulospiral endings.

Answer- a

8. Reciprocal Inhibition is:
   a. the reflex relaxation of the agonist muscle in response to the contraction of the antagonist.
   b. the reflex contraction of the antagonist muscle in response to the contraction of the agonist.
   c. the reflex relaxation of the antagonist muscle in response to the contraction of the agonist.
   d. the reflex relaxation of the muscles as a result of the eccentric movement.

Answer- c

9. The neuromuscular junction is:
   a. a synapse between the terminal end of a motor neuron and a muscle fiber
   b. the junction of two muscle fibers
   c. where an action potential is generated
   d. where the Ca^{++} is stored so that it can be released to the cells to facilitate the firing of the synapse

Answer- a

10. Proprioceptors provide:
    a. feedback concerning pain
    b. feedback concerning the muscles to provide equilibrium
    c. feedback concerning direction of the body
    d. feedback for the visual senses

Answer- b

B. Fill in the Blank

1. Rapid, involuntary response to a stimuli in which a specific stimulus results in a specific motor response is called _____.
Answer- Reflex

2. The reflex relaxation of the antagonist muscle in response to the contraction of the agonist is called _____ _____.
Answer- Reciprocal inhibition

3. _____ _____ is a state of low-level muscle contraction at rest.
Answer- Muscle Tonus

4. _____ is the range of motion in a joint or series of joints that reflects the ability of the musculotendon structures to elongate within the physical limits of the joint.
Answer- Flexibility

5. A form of stretching characterized by an action-reaction bouncing motion in which the joints involved are placed into an extreme range of motion limits by fast active contractions of agonistic muscle groups is called _____ _____.
Answer- Ballistic Stretching

6. A form of stretching in which the muscle to be stretched is slowly put into a position of controlled maximal or near-maximal stretch by contraction of the opposing muscle group and held for 30-60 seconds is called _____ _____.
Answer- Static Stretching

7. _____ is a twitching or spasm in the muscle group that is maximally stretched.
Answer- Myoclonus

8. A stretching technique in which the muscle to be stretched is first contracted maximally. The muscle is then relaxed and is either actively stretched by contraction of the opposing muscle or is passively stretched is called _____ _____.
Answer- Proprioceptive Neuromuscular Facilitation